STRESS

MANAGEMENT

FOR WOMEN

Improve Your Mood to Regain Control of Your Life

(Can Help You to Meditate, Cure Depression and
Enjoy Life Every Day)

Mikel Oliver

Published by Tomas Edwards

© **Mikel Oliver**

All Rights Reserved

Stress Management for Women: Improve Your Mood to Regain Control of Your Life (Can Help You to Meditate, Cure Depression and Enjoy Life Every Day)

ISBN 978-1-990268-28-1

suggested remedies, techniques, or information in this book.

Upon using the information contained in this book, you agree to hold harmless the Author from and against any damages, costs, and expenses, including any legal fees potentially resulting from the application of any of the information provided by this guide. This disclaimer applies to any damages or injury caused by the use and application, whether directly or indirectly, of any advice or information presented, whether for breach of contract, tort, negligence, personal injury, criminal intent, or under any other cause of action.

You agree to accept all risks of using the information presented inside this book. You need to consult a professional medical practitioner in order to ensure you are both able and healthy enough to participate in this program.

Legal & Disclaimer

The information contained in this book is not designed to replace or take the place of any form of medicine or professional medical advice. The information in this book has been provided for educational and entertainment purposes only.

The information contained in this book has been compiled from sources deemed reliable, and it is accurate to the best of the Author's knowledge; however, the Author cannot guarantee its accuracy and validity and cannot be held liable for any errors or omissions. Changes are periodically made to this book. You must consult your doctor or get professional medical advice before using any of the

Table of Contents

Introduction

What happens when we keep "burning the candle" at both ends" until we reach emotional and physical exhaustion? Like the candle itself, we risk burning ourselves out.

There is a parable of a frog sitting in a pot on an oven. If the frog new better, it would likely attempt to get away if it were dropped into a pot of boiling water. Alas, it does not, and the frog does not notice that the water is slowly approaching a boil until its too late and the water reaches an unbearable heat -- at which point it is too hot for the frog to endure.

Have you ever before experienced a sluggish acceptance of the stress around you until whatever is "just way too much," and you can barely function any-longer?

If so, you're not the only one. In 2019 it was reported that approximately 8.3 million adult Americans were reported to have experienced severe emotional distress. The study

revealed that more and more Americans are dealing with stress, anxiety, and depression.

What if we could become aware of distressing indicators earlier, as the frog with the boiling water, and "refuse to enter the water coming to a boil?"

If stress has become one of the most serious health concerns of the 20th century and also a world wide epidemic, then it is time to begin acquiring the tools needed to learn how to properly handle stress.

"Stress is not what happens to us. It's our action TO what takes place. As well as RESPONSE is something we can select." - Maureen Killoran

Attempting to balance the excess stress in our lives, at times, might feel like a difficult task, but it is entirely possible! We all experience excess stress at some stage in our lives.

Many of us have have laid awake at night, thrashing about, not able to sleep, due to unresolved concerns that torture our minds. Most of us say and do things, in the heat of the moment, that we later regret. We get caught up in scenarios that are often beyond our control and leave us really feeling susceptible and upset. We will enjoy greater health and happiness, and much more calm in our lives if we can learn how to handle the excess stress in our lives more effectively.

One of the absolute best ways to keep yourself healthy and happy is to properly manage stress. Stress can have a hugely detrimental influence on an individual's health and happiness. You can choose to either overlook it, and suffer the consequences, or discover ways to overcome stress and find more peace and happiness.

We live in a world of uncertainty, and there's no escaping this truth. All of us experience excess stress at some phase in our lives. And trying to balance that excess stress in our lives, at times, could appear an insurmountable obstacle; but it is attainable!

Now, let's dive into the main purpose of this book and learn how to manage our stress, refocus our stress, and eradicate our stress in healthy ways!

Chapter 1: Acknowledgements

Acknowledgements

I wish to thank every top achiever (165+ of them - I am not naming them all here but you know who you are) who so kindly gave their tips, techniques and expertise during my research.

To my many teachers, trainers and coaches along the journey I salute you all, especially Prof. Adrian Furnham, Sanjay Shah, Tony Burgess and Julie French, and Kash Gill amongst many others.

Having a faith has proven to be a great stress relief for myself so "God... if you are listening... cheers big guy! .... You rock!"

Above all else I must thank the thousands of delegates over the years who have allowed me to test and prove many of the enclosed theories, my amazing friends who put up with me going on and on about my work, and my inspiring wife and son who keep me on the

Why write a book called STRESS MANAGEMENT

Why write a book called STRESS MANAGEMENT

How NOT to be the richest person in the graveyard

... PREVENTION IS THE KEY !!!!

This stress prevention book gives you the tools to increase your certainty, confidence and conviction in managing and preventing levels of stress that otherwise limit your effectiveness. This book is based upon the ways that top achievers think and behave when preventing stress; it looks at the causes and symptoms of stress as well as numerous easy-to-apply methods and processes of stress **prevention**.

Why write a book about stress prevention (and not the management of stress)?

When interviewing top achievers over the past years guess how many of them, when asked the question, "How do you manage your stress?" answered, "Oh yes, I managed my stress"

None of them!

Nearly all of them said, "No,... I do not manage my stress... I prevent it... and this is what I do........". In this book we will therefore look at ways that you can use to identify what causes your stress and what you can do to limit or prevent your levels of stress. We will also be looking at prevention methods including a closed-eye autogenic (a visualized head to toe) relaxation process.

I hope you enjoy this book and reap the benefits of reduced stress, increased effectiveness and increased energy levels. When fully applied you could possibly expect increased levels of alertness, intellectual capacity, thinking power, energy for your personal life and/or energy for your work. Whatever it is you need more energy for, this stress prevention book will make you more effective. The techniques shared within these pages are not designed to "train you" to work with other people and their challenges, but more to help you experiment with numerous simple to use and apply techniques in the hope that you will find one or two things that really work for you.

Causes of Stress

Let's first of all look at and consider just a few of the possible causes of stress. Ask yourself a few quality questions: is there anything you can do to limit or remove the causes of your stress? Where can you begin to look at that? How can you begin to limit, or even remove your stress?

There are so many causes of stress and for each of us, our stressors can be found in different causes and so are very individualized. For example, we could look at your situation and ask does the stress come from home life, personal life, or work? or does it come from a combination of these?

Do you ever feel strained or pressured in any way by one or more of these situations?

For example, at home have you got a newborn baby that is keeping awake at night and into the early hours of morning or maybe you have broken sleep patterns that might be causing you stress?

Maybe you are having a disagreement with a loved one, a friend or a family member that is causing you your stress?

Maybe it is a financial situation (just come into a lot of money or maybe you do not have enough money – either can cause stress) or maybe it is just an unfulfilled life - no sense of purpose?

At work, is it your boss that is screaming at you day in day out about things that are not necessarily your fault? Is it a conflict with other members of staff, clients, suppliers or other members in your team?

Or is it about relationships? Could it be that pets at home are causing you stress? (I used to have a huge friendly, but accident prone Labrador dog that we all loved dearly but boy oh boy did that dog cause us all some stress!!!!!!!).

Is it environment? Are you too hot and you prefer to be cool? Or do you prefer quiet and it's too noisy?

Is it the car?

Is it objects, things, situations, finances, children? What is it for you?

Chapter 2: Working On Your Inner-Self

You can also get effective at fighting stress if you take care of your inner environment. If you are having some internal struggles, that can be another source of stress. Taking some time to resolve some issues within you so that you cultivate a calm inner environment may be the solution you are looking for.

Here are some of the ways you can do this.

8: Practice Mindfulness

You have probably heard before about focusing on the here and now moment in life, right? If you haven't, now you have.

Mindfulness is a practice that allows you to be completely present and focused on where you are and what you are doing. The goal of mindfulness is to make you place less focus on things that are past or those that are to come in future.

The good news is that mindfulness is one of the best techniques I know of that fight stress effectively.

But how does it do this?

Well according to Mindful.org, mindfulness reduces activity in a part of the brain called amygdala. This is the part of the brain that is responsible for producing a stress response in your body. As a result, your stress is reduced.

So how do you practice mindfulness?

The answer to that question can easily take up a book of its own. However, you can simplify it by doing the following:

Whenever you are stressed, take a few moments to observe your breath. Just focus on the in breath and the out breath, making sure to breathe as normally as possible. You can observe how your chest rises and falls when you breathe. Give all your attention to the rising and falling of your chest/stomach, how the air feels as it moves in and out of your mouth/nose, the sounds you make when breathing in and out, the smell of the air etc. Do so as nonjudgmentally as possible. If you notice your mind getting distracted to something else, gently get it back to focusing on your breath. After about 3-5 minutes of focusing on your breath, you will feel relieved and the stress levels will have reduced significantly.

This great article can get you pretty far if you practice what is in it.

9: Practice Meditation

Another effective technique that you can practice to fight stress is meditation.

But what is meditation in the first place?

In simple terms, meditation is a practice that makes your mind focus on one thing such as an object or even your breath. The goal is to promote calmness and mental clarity.

If you are thinking that mindfulness and meditation are closely related, then you are right. In fact, there is a method of meditating that is called mindfulness meditation.

So how is meditation practiced?

Well, likewise meditation is a deep subject that cannot be covered entirely in this book. The subject can best be dedicated to an entire book. If you'd like a personal recommendation from me, you may try reading Meditation for Beginners by Jack Kornfield.

I honestly have to say that meditation is worth all the hype that it gets. Give it a try. You'll be amazed.

10: Repeat Positive Phrases To Yourself

Another fairly effective way of calming your inner-self is by repeating positive phrases to yourself.

"But why does it work?" you may be asking.

Well, Destress.com explains that your thoughts are influenced by what you consistently tell yourself. And in turn, your thoughts affect your actions and the circumstances that arise.

So, if you want to avoid keeping stress in your mind or even prevent the circumstances that lead to stress, then you may want to start by changing what you say to yourself.

How does this work?

It's simple; you can start by telling yourself simple things such as "I am okay. There is nothing to worry about", "Things will turn out well eventually", "It just takes more time, that's all", "What I am doing matters."

I repeat these same phrases every time I feel low and the fact that I am confident enough to tell you about them means I am positive they will work for you as well.

11: Keep A Journal

Keeping a journal can be another powerful way of getting in touch with your inner-self and fighting stress.

The University of Rochester Medical Center reports that getting down on paper what is actually bothering and hurting you helps you fight stress in the following ways:

It helps you identify what triggers your stress and how to control it.

It gives you an opportunity for "talking to yourself" so that you can correct your negative thoughts and behaviors.

It helps you set priorities on what is bothering so that you can get on a path that helps you solve your problems accordingly.

There are many other ways that keeping a journal can help you, but the point is that you realize that keeping one is better for you than doing the opposite.

12: Re-Invent Your Values

You can also keep stress away by taking a hard look at what you choose to believe and value.

Examine your beliefs and replace what isn't working for you.

We are a society that tends to adopt the values of others without questioning. The truth is; you can do yourself some good by being somewhat different from the crowd.

For instance, I have people within my social circle who spend well beyond their means, and end up paying the price. Does this mean that I should behave the same way even when I see that it's clearly putting them in a hole? No.

You should do the same.

Take some time and ask yourself this; "Am I doing this because everyone is doing or because it makes perfect sense to me and is in line with what I truly believe?"

For instance, creating your own definition of success can go a long way in ensuring you put less pressure on yourself as you try to measure up to societal values. And this can help relieve some of your stress.

I hope that by now, you have some good ideas that can help you work on your inner-self.

Next up, we will be looking at how adopting a tough mindset can help you fight stress.

Chapter 3: Types Of Stress

Acute stress. Have you ever noticed that when you are stuck in traffic and your anxiety is high, your focus gets sharper and you think only of the task at hand? This is your stress response kicking in, giving you the mental clarity and focus needed to deal with a lifethreatening situation. It may not be actually life threatening, but your body may think so. Episodes of acute stress tend to string together. Think about stressors at home, work and in your social life. While these things are individually taxing, together, they add up to low level chronic stress. Learning to handle these individual situations in a more healthy way can decrease overall chronic stress. Chronic stress is something we all feel every day. It is the result of the alarm clock going off, getting the kids ready for school and fighting traffic to get to work on time. Small moments of stress are needed to get your body in gear and boost energy to focus on the task at hand. Most people are under a veil of chronic stress all day long. The body responds to stress in a number of ways. First, it releases adrenaline, frequently called the body's ‚stress hormone'. It is released by the adrenal glands to raise the heart rate, blood pressure and shortens breath to take in more oxygen for the body to use. The response goes back to our primal instincts. The body needs to prepare to run from danger, or stand and fight, the so-called ‚fight or flight' response. Cortisol is another stress hormone that is expressed with adrenaline. While a little cortisol once in a while is a good thing, persistent exposure to cortisol, like with several small episodes of chronic stress, has some negative effects on the body. It increases blood sugar, which can lead to diabetes over time. It decreases thyroid function, cognitive function and immune system support after prolonged bouts of stress. The most advertised impact of cortisol is its ability to store excess belly fat. When the body thinks its survival is at stake, it will take measures to store as much energy in fat as it can. Stubborn belly fat is a common symptom of chronic stress. The adrenal glands themselves can also be affected. Adrenal fatigue happens when the glands are forced to produce excessive amounts of adrenaline, cortisol and other stress hormones as a response to stress. Over time, too little hormones are made and the body suffers from extreme fatigue, slowing metabolism and suppressed immune system. As this continues, overall mood and attitude become affected. You become more irritable, less able to focus, and it becomes increasingly more difficult to deal with minor stresses. It will become difficult to sleep, leaving you more fatigued during the day. The less energy you have, the more susceptible you are to stress. It is a vicious circle that can only be stopped by eliminating the source of the problem, your stress levels. The only way to stop these negative effects is to decrease overall amounts of stress in your life. While avoiding it completely is not always possible, eliminating some sources of stress and learning to cope with unavoidable stress in a healthy way will reward you with better health overall. Hopefully the stress of hearing about what causes stress will be the prompt you need to work on management. From here on out, we will focus on ways to deal with everyday situations in a meaningful way that reduces stress. First off, it is important to recognize possible stressors in your life. They can come from a number of places, or from one thing in particular. Common problems people face are the following:

• Family life-difficult extended family members, children and spouses can test your patience on a daily basis. While a particular person may not be the problem, making sure everyone is happy and taken care of and where they need to be can be a stressful daily task.

• Health-declining and health are a major concern. There may not be anything you can do about your own health, or that of a loved one, and that causes anxiety for the future.

• Money-worrying about paying bills and making ends meet plagues most people. Money is the key to keeping a roof over your head and food on the table.

• Work-getting along with co-workers plus increasingly demanding jobs and deadlines often push stress levels through the roof. Not to mention the stress of commuting to and from work in heavy traffic.

• Chores and household duties. If there seems to be a never ending pile of dirty laundry and dishes, you're not alone. There will always be chores to be done, and keeping on top of them can be taxing.

Chapter 4: Effects Of Stress On Your Health And Body

There is no question about it that stress can majorly affect your health in a negative way but stress can also have consequences on your body too. So if you teach yourself how to recognize stress symptoms on time, so that will only give you an advantage on how to manage stress itself.

If you neglect any of the common stress symptoms that can cause you some serious health problems such as various heart diseases, obesity, diabetes, high blood pressure, asthma, depression, anxiety, arthritis, skin conditions, and headaches.

Your regular heart rate is increased which is not such a good thing obviously, and your breathing becomes shallow and faster than usual, blood pressure level increases drastically also you start feeling muscle tension all over your body and you find it hard to relax even for a moment.

Around 85% of all visits to the doctor are because of stress related issues than can developed into something much worse. There are extremely numerous physical and emotional disorders that are related to stress and can easily disturb your immune system which can lead to various infections that you probably wouldn't contract if you took precautionary measures on time. So the sooner you accept stress as a part of your life and start treating it like one, the better.

How to avoid, relieve and manage Stress

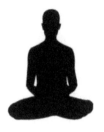

MEDITATE

When stress makes you nervous and anxious one of the possibilities to reduce stress is considering meditation, even if you only spend a couple of minutes during the day to meditate it can still calm you and help you find your inner peace. Meditation can be done by anyone and it's totally free so you don't have to buy some fancy equipment in order to help you relax your mind. Also one of the greatest advantages of meditation is that you can practice it anywhere and at any given time. Meditation is practiced for thousands of years already so if it's still practiced today by millions all over the world, that proves it as an efficient method for finding yourself and restoring a piece of mind on your own, and I definitely recommend meditation as one of the techniques in managing stress.

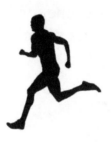

EXERCISE

Starting to exercise can lift your spirit back up in no time. Exercising can improve your mood drastically and it will also boost your self-confidence because physical activity produces endorphin in your brain which is a feel-good hormone and it automatically reduces stress levels and anxiety. The feeling that you are actually doing something productive and positive for your body can go a long way in ling term stress management. But this doesn't mean that you have to suddenly start exercising like crazy, in fact you should start slow and "learn how to walk before you are able to fly" start increasing the level of physical activity gradually and not all at once because it can actually be harmful if you overdo it so take one step at a time in order to extract the maximum benefits of exercising.

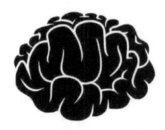

THINK POSITIVELY

You should practice telling yourself that you will only do the things in life that suits you and not let negative thoughts to overwhelm you when you are not feeling so good. Stop beating yourself over something that happened recently or in the past that went wrong because you only increasing the stress for nothing since worrying about stuff that you can't change is completely unnecessary you should forgive yourself for your benefit and move on by focusing on the present and what you can do to better yourself. No matter how hard things are right now, remember that it could always be worst, so be grateful for what you have and who you are. Learn from your past mistakes and make sure to not repeat them, use them as an advantage in your life because even if they were mistakes you could still learn something from them. Give yourself some credit for a recent small or big success that you had, believe that you can succeed and you will. Using positive words when you are talking to someone can subconsciously improve your state of mind.

LAUGH

You probably heard this line a hundred

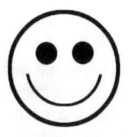

times in your life but it's true (Laughter is the best medicine) that is only a saying but laughter can improve your immune system because it relieves physical tension and stress, and can relax your muscles for at

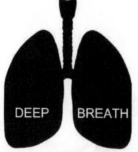

least one hour after a good hearty laugh. Laughter also increases blood flow and improves the function of blood vessels which protects your heart from cardiovascular issues.

BREATHE

You can practice deep breathing where ever you are, just straighten your back, close your eyes and inhale through your nose deeply and exhale through your mouth letting out as much air as you can repeat this for about ten times and you will instantly fell a difference. Repeat this exercise at least once every day and you will definitely improve your feeling overall.

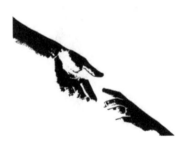

REACH OUT

Read similar stories to yours online, connect with people, because you're definitely not alone even if everything seems like you are. Reading about similar struggles like the one you're going through at the moment can help you gain perspective and learn from other people's mistakes before you make them on your own. You will probably find optimistic stories that were worse than yours but came out well at the end. Find a friend online or in real life that goes through the same thing and pull inspiration from one another as you go along the way of improving yourself. Join support groups because there is nothing like the ability to talk about what is bothering you with people that understand what you're going through.

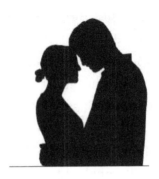

EXPRESS YOUR FEELINGS

Hugging and telling your loved ones how much you love them once in a while even for no apparent reason whatsoever can always have a positive feedback on your mood and reduce stress, because when you interact with people that mean something to you, your brain releases the hormone of happiness endorphin and it can instantly make you feel better as well as the person that you are interacting with. And knowing that you made your loved one feel good, it will naturally make you feel better too.

YOGA

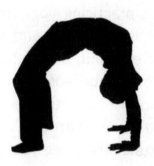

Practicing Yoga can benefit your physical and mental health and can help you manage stress and anxiety on daily basis. Combining yoga with meditation can reduce risk of chronic diseases connected to heart and high blood pressure issues. It can also reduce physical pain in any part of your body and will definitely help you sleep better at night, as well as improve tour flexibility and balance. There are many different types of yoga and you can choose the one that is best for you, in my opinion the best yoga type for stress relief for me is Hatha Yoga which is the most practiced type of yoga in America and it combines body postures with breathing techniques for having a peaceful mind. Always wear loose and comfortable clothes when practicing yoga and all you need for this, is a flat floor and a bit space so you can stretch out. Don't practice yoga with a full stomach because that can result in unwanted situations so it's recommended to wait at least three hours before you start stretching yourself to the limits of your body.

READ

A good book that can take you away in a fantasy world so you can escape reality for a while is a perfect way to get your thoughts of your everyday problems that are bothering you and causing stress. Even if you never liked fantasy and science fiction books, you should give them a chance maybe it will be a pleasant surprise, but if you still don't want to read a fantasy book, then the best choice would be a comedy genre so you can have a laugh, and we all know that laughter can only be a good thing.

NO

LEARN TO SAY NO

Always trying to be helpful and saying yes all the time isn't healthy, so you must learn how to say –**NO**- to people once in a while. I know that it can be hard to say No and risking of hurting someone's feelings but you have to do it in order to help yourself in becoming a better and more respected person. Don't think if you say yes to your colleagues always when they ask you for a favor will make them respect you or having a good opinion for you just because you never said no to them, because people can often think even less of you when you agree to any given task that they ask you to do, and some of them will even exploit a person that always goes their way. Just because every year you were the one to write the business plan of the company you work for, doesn't mean that you always have to do it. Just say No and use that time to pursue something new, something else that you like, or even just take the time to relax and enjoy.

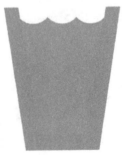

DRINK MORE WATER

Don't underestimate the power of drinking water since every organ in our body and even our brain needs water in order to function properly. You should make sure to drink at least 5 glasses of clean water per day because it will detoxify your body which automatically means a healthier body, and that also means a healthier mind. Drinking clean water regularly, can help you lose some extra weight and if you decide to exercise on top of that, you will be proud of the final results. Having a healthier body will increase your confidence and with that reduce stress along the way which is what we want after all.

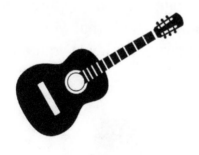

TRY NEW THINGS

Find a hobby if you already don't have one, and even if you do have hobbies you should always try new things that you always wanted but never had the time for it. Maybe you should learn how to play a guitar or any other instrument because music can be a huge stress antidote. Do something fun that you normally wouldn't do, experiment with new subjects in your life, set your mind on one thing and don't stop until you achieve it, start with a small thing and don't give up. When you actually achieve something that you've planned and do it successfully, you will realize that there is almost nothing that you can't do with the right mindset and positive thinking. If you think that you can do it, **YOU CAN**. Start believing in your abilities.

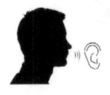

DO NOT LISTEN TO GOSSIP OR GOSSIP YOURSELF

Nothing good can come from gossiping, if you gossip you can only lose your credibility in the eyes of your loved ones or even society in general, even if you think that gossiping about bad people is ok, it's not because when people notice that you care about someone else's problems, they automatically assume that you are not a trust worthy person which can result in bad credibility and affect your work and life progress as an individual in general. So keep in mind to just mind your own business all the time because it's clearly better to look for new ways in making your life better than thinking and stressing yourself over someone else's life issues.

RESPECT YOURSELF

Take time just for yourself every day, even if it's just 5 or 10 minutes to think about what you want in life and are you currently happy with what you're doing and who you are with. You must respect yourself so others can follow, but you also need to give respect in order to get respect from the people in your surroundings.

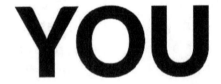

YOU

Chapter 5: Symptoms Of Anxiety

Anxiety manifests itself in a variety of symptoms, including the following:

-Sweating
-Nausea
-Churning stomach
-Muscle tenseness
-Feeling numb in your legs, arms, or hands
-Headaches
-Backaches
-Trembling
-Diarrhea
-Fast heartbeat
-Thoughts that don't go away
-Restlessness
-Avoiding things, places, or people
-Compulsions
-Faintness

Some other signs that you might have anxiety are having habitually negative thought patterns like: catastrophizing, personalization, and "all or nothing" thinking. Catastrophizing or worst-case-scenario thinking is when you blow ordinary events out of proportion. Personalization is when you take an event too personally when it has nothing to do with you. It also involves feeling out of control, victimized, or helpless in a given situation. All or nothing thinking is characterized by viewing a situation in one of two extremes, as always happening or never happening. If a person uses the words "always" or "never," this is often a sign that they could have this thought pattern.

Understanding the Stress Response

Your body has a default biological response to stressors. Some people refer to the stress response as the fight-or-flight response.

When the flight-or-flight response is activated, it has the following physical signs:
-dilated   pupils
-heightened   alertness
-increased   heart   rate

-pale or clammy skin (caused by constricted blood vessels in the skin and sweat glands)
-less blood flow in the digestive system
-more blood flow in the arm and leg muscles

Let's slow down the process, however, to understand what happens at each step of the response. The stress response process begins when you encounter a threat in the environment. This could be as ordinary as a car cutting you off on the highway or receiving a phone call from a person you are having a conflict with. Your body responds to this threat by activating your hypothalamus, an area at the base of your brain. The hypothalamus sends hormone signals to the adrenal glands which in turn release the hormones called cortisol and adrenaline. At healthy levels, these hormones are helpful for your body. Cortisol increases glucose in your blood to boost brain activity and physical responsiveness. Adrenaline increases blood pressure and speeds up your heart rate which results in a heightened source of energy. Once the threat is over, your body returns to a calmer condition. Heart rate slows down to its normal rate and cortisol and adrenaline levels drop.

The fight-or-flight response also relates to anxiety since those with an anxiety disorder experience a triggering of their stress response when there is no threat or danger present in a given situation. According to the Depression and Bipolar Support Alliance, people that have anxiety tend to have a more overactive stress response than the average person.

But back to the fight-or-fliught response. If this process is a good thing, why are we even talking about it? Well, the fight-or-flight response becomes a concern when it is activated for a long period of time. The body's stress response was meant for short-term stresses, to help humans survive and escape difficult scenarios by either fighting or running away. In the 21st century world, due to technology and the high level of comfort Western society has, our biological stress response can be more harmful than helpful in the average person's life.

Long-term exposure to stress hormones like cortisol and adrenaline can disrupt your body's natural functions and they increase your risk for sickness and disease. Some of these negative problems are: depression, heart disease, weight gain, anxiety, sleep problems, poor memory and/or concentration, and digestive problems.

Some additional signs of high cortisol and adrenaline levels are:
-Catching colds easily
-Having a low libido
-Gaining abdominal weight (which can be a sign of too much cortisol)
-Feeling tired, even after getting 8 or more hours of sleep
-Frequent back pain and/or headaches

Chapter 6: The Power Of Prayer

The prayer to be a positive mental exercise, something that lets you talk out your fears, feel better about a bad situation, etc. Those are true as well!

However, the power of prayer goes even deeper than that. I was raised in a religious family as a member of the Church of Jesus Christ of Latter-Day Saints. When I was in middle school, I started to seriously reflect, ponder and work out if in reality what I had been taught as a child was really true and something I wanted to dedicate my life too. More specifically I wanted to know if someone was actually listening to me pray day and night, does God really exist and would he answer me? Needless to say, I decided to get on my knees and pray, with real intent, or in other words, ready to follow whatever answer I received.

I stand as a witness that God answered my prayer. Not a vision or a voice of any sort but an unmistakable answer that I was being listened to, that he loved me and that I knew what I had been taught as a child was true.

That experience along with countless others have demonstrated to me that there is real and tangible power in reaching out to the Supreme Being that always is reaching out to you. Never hesitate to pray! Because there is a God I know that Satan is real and he does not want us to be happy or have the support of a loving God.

If nothing else, follow James's council in the New Testament, James 1:5. You lose nothing by connecting to the Lord but stand to gain everything.

However I no longer doubt prayer's effectiveness. I just doubt I was praying for the right things. Once I had my life-changing experience and found God and knew him for myself, I became utterly convinced of his existence as well as convinced of some things about religion.

One is prayer. The primary purpose of prayer is to put us in communion with our soul, with the universe, with God, with all of those as a whole. In this state, we can communicate easily with ourselves and we can ask for what we really need and be sure of getting it. If we ask. And if we ask for what we really need and not what we think we want. And tell ourselves the truths we need to hear. "I am loved. I deserve to be loved. I will do good things for myself. I will help myself." Affirmations and guided meditation is another form of prayer. Try to talk to your deepest self and change what it believes. To be truly effective though, we need to know exactly what we're afraid of and exactly what we need to hear to motivate us.

I have evidence of the power of self-talk. I am getting happier as a result of remembering to tell myself good things and doing good things for myself.

One way to think about it is that God is the light. He shines love down on all of us to help us live and thrive.

In the most general sense, prayer is an act of worship that seeks to activate a rapport with the divine through deliberate communication, and this may or may not include an invocation in the process. Either way, the act of praying has been an essential part of what it means to be human for quite a while. There is a longstanding mystical tradition of praying which dates back tens of thousands of years. As part of this ancient legacy of devotion, I have prayed with my father and he with his, and so on and so forth, all the way back to the first recognition of divinity nearly four thousand generations ago.

Granted, depending on how and why people pray, the act itself might either be individual or communal and could take place in public or in private. There really is no limit to the different kinds of spirituality and religiosity that can emerge. In regards to this, spirituality is for the soul while religiosity is for God. To better understand what I mean by this it's important to realize that a long time ago all of the indigenous people on the habitable continents were animists. This formed the basis of their spirituality. So, from their point of view communication with both embodied and disembodied souls was essential to their way of life. As a result of this, in line with the customs of their local tribe, a shaman would enter trance states in an effort to gain better access to metaphysical space. Then, religiosity eventually grew out of that spirituality. This inevitably gave rise to countless different creation myths among early humans.

Dozens of millennia later, monotheism has become the dominant form of both spirituality and religiosity in the world. However, the act of praying has evolved and it will continue to do so as the soul improves over time. God only knows what we might do next. For now, observant Jews currently pray three times a day, with lengthier sessions on certain occasions, such as the Shabbat and during the reading of the Torah. Then again, in yet another example of the Abrahamic faiths, the command to ritual prayer is mentioned in several of the Surahs in the Qur'an. Prayer is absolutely vital to Muslims. In the religion of Islam there are five daily obligatory prayers that are required for Salat which is one of the five pillars of their faith.

Meanwhile, Hindus have a very different form of worship. Regardless, as part of their religion, once a year in India tens of millions of devotees of several Eastern traditions come together in the largest congregation on the planet. There, at the confluence of three sacred rivers where Sadhus sit smoking Ganja, people of all ages celebrate their faith together as one. This incredibly holy festival currently consists of the biggest prayer group on Earth. Although in all likelihood the Muslims will hold the record in the not-too-distant future. As another of the five pillars of their faith, the Hajj is an annual pilgrimage to Mecca that has been drawing a bigger crowd with each passing year and the trend shows no signs of slowing down anytime soon. Enormous congregations like this are magnificent achievements for humanity, either way. More importantly, they offer us glimpses of the kind of overwhelmingly glorious global piety that our species could one day achieve.

Now, don't get me wrong, it's really important for everyone to understand that this isn't just about doing something at certain times, or in special places, in tremendously spectacular ways. That's not really the point at all, although those things are still very important. Instead, occasions such as those should serve as reminders for us to always live with a positive spiritual and religious attitude. With that in mind, the act of saying grace before meals is something everyone might want to do just as an easy way to incorporate God into what they already do on a daily basis. No matter what, the point is that it's very important for everyone to make room for the Supreme Being in their lives. Ultimately, prayer is simply about making yourself available to God, while at the same time making God available to you.

The power of prayer should not be underestimated.

"The prayer of a righteous man is powerful and effective. Elijah was a man just like us. He prayed earnestly that it would not rain, and it did not rain on the land for three and a half years. Again he prayed, and the heavens gave rain, and the earth produced its crops." God most definitely listens to prayers, answers prayers, and moves in response to prayers.

Jesus taught, "...I tell you the truth, if you have faith as small as a mustard seed, you can say to this mountain, 'Move from here to there' and it will move. Nothing will be impossible for you"

"The weapons we fight with are not the weapons of the world. On the contrary, they have divine power to demolish strongholds. We demolish arguments and every pretension that sets itself up against the knowledge of God, and we take captive every thought to make it obedient to Christ." The Bible urges us, "And pray in the Spirit on all occasions with all kinds of prayers and requests. With this in mind, be alert and always keep on praying for all the saints"

Power Of Prayer - How do I tap into it?

The power of prayer is not the result of the person praying. Rather, the power resides in the God who is being prayed to.

"This is the confidence we have in approaching God: that if we ask anything according to his will, he hears us. And if we know that he hears us - whatever we ask - we know that we have what we asked of him." No matter the person praying, the passion behind the prayer, or the purpose of the prayer - God answers prayers that are in agreement with His will. His answers are not always yes, but are always in our best interest. When our desires line up with His will, we will come to understand that in time. When we pray passionately and purposefully, according to God's will, God responds powerfully!

We cannot access powerful prayer by using "magic formulas." Our prayers being answered is not based on the eloquence of our prayers. We don't have to use certain words or phrases to get God to answer our prayers. In fact, Jesus rebukes those who pray using repetitions, "And when you pray, do not keep on babbling like pagans, for they think they will be heard because of their many words. Do not be like them, for your Father knows what you need before you ask him"

Prayer is communicating with God. All you have to do is ask God for His help.

"Then they cried out to the LORD in their trouble, and he brought them out of their distress. He stilled the storm to a whisper; the waves of the sea were hushed. They were glad when it grew calm, and he guided them to their desired haven." There is power in prayer!

Power Of Prayer - For what kind of things should I pray?

God's help through the power of prayer is available for all kinds of requests and issues. "Do not be anxious about anything, but in everything, by prayer and petition, with thanksgiving, present your requests to God. And the peace of God, which transcends all understanding, will guard your hearts and your minds in Christ Jesus."

The Lord's prayer is not a prayer we are supposed to memorize and simply recite to God. It is only an example of how to pray and the things that should go into a prayer - worship, trust in God, requests, confession, protection, etc. Pray for these kinds of things, but speak to God using your own words.

The Word of God is full of accounts describing the power of prayer in various situations. The power of prayer has overcome enemies, conquered death.

God, through prayer, opens eyes, changes hearts, heals wounds, and grants wisdom The power of prayer should never be underestimated because it draws on the glory and might of the infinitely powerful God of the universe!

"All the peoples of the earth are regarded as nothing. He does as he pleases with the powers of heaven and the peoples of the earth. No one can hold back his hand or say to him: 'What have you done?'"

Chapter 7: Think To Decrease Stress

Stress is reduced by thinking, and you like life more. Is your glass half-full or half-empty? The way you answer that question illustrates your overall outlook and how well you deal with stress. But thinking goes beyond being a stress buster. Studies indicate it reduces your likelihood of melancholy, increases your life span, and enables you to take care of hardships in a better way. However, an attitude does not mean that you embrace Emu-like qualities and keep your head in the sand and ignore the causes of stress or problems. All about coming events in a manner, It's! Adopting a positive attitude can be difficult if Stress is feeling down or bombards you.

The Power Of Positive Thinking

Optimism's Advantages extend past stress relief to Health, productivity, and more rewarding relationships.

Individuals with a positive outlook tend to encounter:

Reduced prevalence of depression

Lower stress levels and therefore are better able to deal with stress-causing occasions

A heightened life span

Overall greater health

Enhanced psychological well-being

People with a positive outlook in life are more likely to smoke, and to live a healthier lifestyle and drink less alcohol.

Positive Thoughts And Dealing With Stress

The definition of fear says the way. We perceive a situation that could affect our ability and our stress levels to deal with stress. In a brief....the manner, you think affects the amount of Stress you feel! There have been scientific study Andrews and colleagues (2008) that demonstrated that when people who reported using a joyful mood (positive ideas) had reduced levels of the stress hormone cortisol. Optimists tend to blame their failures Circumstances, and if they do fail, they often get a "try again" mindset. Optimists are more likely to possess problem-orientated Coping strategies. On the other hand, pessimists are more likely to blame Failure and therefore are reluctant to "give it a try" again together with the adverse experience. Pessimists are more likely to prevent coping or to be in denial with stress.

What's Positive Thinking?

That Is, positive thinking is psychological and a psychological of expecting results attitude. It does not mean that you dismiss the negativity and find the world in pink. It suggests that your strategy unpleasant constructively and positively.

A Lot of People confuse thinking that is optimistic with optimistic blindness. Where a desirable behavior to the difficulty is prioritized, thinking relies on a vital approach.

Research has demonstrated that the consequences of thinking Extend beyond stress management. Numerous positive results include but Aren't Limited to:

Less depression and stress

Improved psychological equilibrium

Better capacity to handle stress and stress-causing occasions

Better health and improved lifespan

Healthier and more robust relationships

Greater productivity

The general feeling of joy

Among those theories why the health benefits are felt by Peoples Since with a favorable mindset enables people to deal with stressful circumstances, which, consequently, reduces the effects of strain on the health. If they exercise, thinking is.

How To Decrease Stress Through Positive Thinking Distinct Procedures

A Good Deal of Individuals Believes that they start practicing Positive will have ideas. Well, it's not perfect. Thoughts are a part of our brain works. It's entirely natural to have negative ideas. About minding those ideas that are negative once and for all, positive thinking isn't. It's all about understanding how to handle when those ideas look in the mind of one. The very first step towards practicing positive thinking is identifying contradictory ideas. Individuals who believe often magnify the unwanted Aspects of a scenario and filter out all of the positive ones. Another quality of thinkers that are unwanted is your capacity to assume that the challenge is inside them and to customize the issues. Watch things, and they tend to expect the worst if something happens. Should you find yourself, you are a thinker. Admitting it is the first step towards thinking. It's time As Soon as you know, your Method of thinking To make attempts to take a look at things. The way to implement it?

Change Your Negative Thoughts To Positive Ones

Allowing dreams to hang around for a while triggers Stress and depression.

That's why it's necessary to respond to contrary ideas.

Here are a Few Tips to Help you deal with your negativity:

Favorable Affirmations: positive self-talk helps change negative ideas into positive, beneficial affirmations. Rather than saying, "I made a mistake," you could try, "This is a chance for me to understand." It doesn't mean the issue is neglected by that you. It doesn't restrict yourself and means that you give it a chance.

Favorable Visualization: once we imagine a circumstance, we are apt to see more chances for discovering ways to fix problems. So the next time you utilize, attempt to visualize the event. It can allow you to handle your stress and find answers to bring your ideas.

Favorable individuals and Occasions: positive thinking has a more significant effect once we surround ourselves with positive people and occasions. They have an immediate impact on the mood. So a small positivity will not hurt you. On the contrary, it is going to improve your motivation to practice thinking.

Know And Use Your Strengths Daily

Using and Understanding our strengths helps us become happier and more optimistic about being productive in the office and be satisfied with life generally, about ourselves. But studies show that not even one from 3 people could name their strengths. Strength-awareness helps to comprehend our skills and the ways we can leverage them. This, in turn, promotes self-esteem and self-confidence. When we understand what we can utilize and are useful in Optimistic thinking, lives grow potential. It will become a necessity.

So the way to identify Best strengths?

Utilizing strengths tests: asset evaluations will be the best way to find out the best character traits of one. I have been advocated a strengths finder. It's known as HIGH5 and helps research how it is possible to use these strengths more efficiently and identify the top five strengths.

Asking friends and coworkers: of discovering the best abilities of one, another method is by asking colleagues and friends. Their view can allow you to comprehend the purposes of using your strengths and also the areas.

Consulting with a mentor: development professionals and career coaches may steer you on your quest for high personality traits and strengths.

Practice, Practice, Practice

Many people don't adopt thinking Want results. They turn their backs when change doesn't occur immediately. This kind of person typically constitutes the vast majority of people who don't accept favorable thinking. Well, this is your key. Positive thinking won't turn you in person that is positive immediately and doesn't do magic. It's an ongoing process of practicing the tactics mentioned above rather than giving up. It is similar to learning a new language. Nobody is capable of renovating French one day. The same logic functions for positive thinking. For the mind to turn negative thinking patterns, it requires a great deal of practice and time. It's all about using actions to change those and figuring out how to recognize negative thoughts. Thinking isn't the energy of altering The hostile world to a pink one that is favorable. It's a mindset that can help handle situations that are adverse by adopting a positive attitude, which helps deal with the stress associated with those scenarios that are negative.

Reframe

Consider how to reduce and manage stress in your life by considering specific circumstances that are stressful. Reframing is a mechanism that entails a focus on a situation's advantages. Think about reframing, so you are the hero as telling your story. This requires distance, particularly when the problem is currently attempting or has powerful feelings attached to it. Once you have space, you've got the liberty. A good illustration is my morning commute. Days among my four Kids will have somewhat late running. I am somebody who prides me, and this felt vulnerable to me. Rather than continuing to think thoughts of the behind, I chose to tell a story to myself. In my account, I was being protected by the world I would have had when I wished to leave if I'd left. Is this accurate? Possibly. I don't understand what could have happened if we'd left, but when it might help me to feel a bit less nervous about my lateness, the reframe proved to be a stress relief.

Posting

A sign out front boasts A Place for Miracles, and the had been miraculous. We had been taught to utilize whenever the procedure for stress management ideas or a sense happened to us. You are not necessarily readily available to reflect in your thought process every time a negative, stressful, or embarrassing idea arises but by building a post, a little notation in a laptop or your smartphone, you can return later in the day or first thing in the morning when you feel relaxed and calm and require a more in-depth look at the reason why you're feeling stressed.

Utilize a Collection of Questions like:

What were you feeling?

Where did you feel within your body for it?

What did you think would happen if you did not believe that?

Reflections and these articles can lead one to understand why you pick the ideas you select, and this, in turn, permits you to replace these ideas (assuming they're no longer serving you). Frequently a one is replaced by a notion that is half-full.

Mindfulness

Spending some time is another way your thinking. Individuals who spend time in meditation benefit the capacity and the ability to begin according to a practice of focusing on a mantra or the breath; there are distractions of thoughts, feelings, or sensations, and beginning. I visit the Dalai Lama laughing or grinning; I'm reminded that a brain that's spent some time is primed for pleasure.

Growing Or Gain Mindset

Carol Dweck has been famous for her research. She identified two kinds of mindsets--expansion and mended. Having a mindset, you're born with intellect or talent, and it is. Using an increase mindset, no matter IQ or ability, it is possible to become on the flip side. Specialist Ash Buchanan has an additional advantage mindset to this particular mix. An advantage mindset assembles on a development mindset, although you attempt to meet your potential, but opt to do it in a manner which serves all's well-being. Optimistic thinking is a by-product when you decide to come up with again or growth mindset. You quit become receptive to the possibility of limitless potential and seeing possible depending on your genetics. You have when that is done for the greater good.

Self-Compassion

A Fantastic spot to plant the seeds of thinking is with self-compassion. When you begin taking minutes to clinic self-care, you lower your stress levels based on self-compassion (in adolescents) researcher Karen Bluth, that utilizes touch--like putting hands on your heart, softly stroking your cheek, or depriving yourself to elicit hormones such as oxytocin that encourage positive emotions. Look at using a quotation to Begin off with a favorable attitude. A daily dose of pleasure may set the tone for positive thinking. Attempt a minute of gratitude to seal the joys. Based on Barbara Fredrickson, a favorable psychologist and writer of Positivity: "The great number of research other scientists and I have run positivity is poised to stay only interesting dinner conversation till you deepen your self-study. Toward what works for you, and you want to pivot away from what's worked for others. Have your eureka!' moments. Discover for yourself precisely what rouses real and heartfelt positivity."

Surround Yourself With Additional Positive Individuals

If you believe you are getting an optimist takes practice. Transforming a habit of thinking won't happen. However, with practice, you can create your thinking, which your outlook will enhance, encourage connections, And lower your stress. You are surrounding yourself Perpetuates of believing, which makes it challenging to modify your custom. Attempt to surround yourself with others so that you model and learn their Believing in unique scenarios.

Chapter 8: Preventing Stress

Avoiding stress, anxiety, and worry is arguably the best way to keep yourself protected from its harms.

Let's look at some of the easiest ways to prevent, alleviate or eliminate some of life's common stressors.

Become Better at Time Management

A lot of stress comes from a lack of good time management skills. Poor time management skills leads us to waste time on meaningless tasks. Do you miss work deadlines? Do you find it difficult or impossible to juggle your personal and professional responsibilities? Do you ever have time to just relax?

Lack of consistent and productive time management skills starts a snowball effect on your stress level because time management is part of everyday life both personally and professionally.

Create To-Do Lists

Because of the absence of To-do lists, we often forget to tend to important tasks on time and sometimes forget to do anything at all. To prevent the stress that comes from forgetting or avoiding important tasks, make a habit of preparing your To-do list for the next day the night before. Place that To-do list on an important wall or place in your home and make a soft-copy of it in your phone and laptop too so that you are aware of all your important tasks.

Prioritize Your Work

The inability to prioritize work is one of the major causes of poor time management skills. When you cannot distinguish between meaningful and meaningless tasks, you will either find yourself directing your focus to unproductive and meaningless tasks or lacking focus entirely.

When preparing your To-do list, determine your high priority tasks. High priority tasks are tasks that increase your productivity, help you reach your goals fast, and ultimately bring you peace of mind.

Once you are aware of your high priority tasks, put them first on your To-do list and attend to them first. Regularly evaluate your personal, professional, health and relationship goals so you can figure out the high priority tasks that can help you accomplish those goals fast. For instance, if your health related goal is to build more muscle mass, a high priority task relevant to it would be to increase your protein intake.

Once you start doing the high priority tasks first, you will accomplish a lot more in less time, which will help you prevent stressful situations.

Do One Thing at a Time

Contrary to popular belief, multi-tasking does not help you manage your time efficiently. In fact, it does just the opposite. When you try to do too many things at once, you lose focus on the important tasks. When you focus on too many tasks, the quality of your completed tasks will suffer and you will end up wasting time instead of making good use of it. To ensure this does not happen to you, do one thing at a time.

Whenever you have to work on a task, attend to only that and nothing else. Focus on the reasons why that task is important for you and keep recalling these reasons so you can stay focused on the present task. It can be difficult to avoid distraction and if you're like me, it will take time and practice to keep your focus.

Avoid Paying Attention to Your Distractions

The numerous distractions around us are often the reasons we cannot concentrate on important chores. If you notice yourself multi-tasking too often or often pushing back important chores, it is likely because you have allowed the many distractions around you to sidetrack you. Spend some quality time alone and think of all the things that distract you from your work.

Once you have figured those out, look for ways to avoid them.

If you feel tempted to play games on your phone each time you sit to work on an office project, switch off your phone and get working. If you feel the urge to sleep when it is time to start an important task, incentivize yourself to begin that task by setting an attractive reward to it.

Reward yourself each time you attend to your important tasks first and make good use of your time so you become motivated to do this frequently.

Complete Your Pending Chores First

"Much of the stress that people feel doesn't come from having too much to do. It comes from not finishing what they've started." – David Allen

If you have any pending chores that are threatening your emotional wellbeing, attend to them right away even if their deadlines have passed.

When you finish those tasks, you will enjoy a sense of fulfillment and will know that you can indeed complete your tasks. This encourages you to tend to other tasks and get work done on time to avert the stress that comes from deferring your tasks.

Try these time management hacks to avert the storm of stress that is trying to make its way into your life.

Improve Your Lifestyle

The decisions you make about your life and the different choices you opt for directly affect your emotional well-being and stress levels. A lot of stress in our lives comes from living an unhealthy lifestyle.

To ensure you avoid stress, you have to improve your lifestyle. Here are a few ways to live a healthy lifestyle that helps you prevent stress.

Have a Clear Direction and Sense of Purpose

A lack of a clear direction and not having a sense of purpose are often the indirect reasons behind a stressful life. When you do not have meaningful goals or goals to attend to, or do not know which direction you are heading, you are likely to pay more attention to unimportant tasks. To make sure that uneasiness does not turn into chronic stress, find your true sense of purpose in life.

Give yourself the gift of time and focus on what you want. Think of what gives your life meaning. Is your family what matters the most to you, or are you a strong, independent individual who is fulfilled from work related activities?

Find out if different spheres of your life such as health, wealth, love, happiness, relationships, spirituality, profession etc. are heading in the right direction. Ask yourself questions like, "What do I really want to do with my life?" "How can I make the most of my life?" "Is what I am doing the right way to live my life?" "What truly makes me feel happy and content?"

These questions will help you figure out your purpose in life and build meaningful goals around it so you get clarity on how you aim to live your life.

Live a Balanced Life

Striking a balance between your work, personal, health, and family demands and needs is an important part of keeping stress at bay. Think of the adage "All work and no play makes Jack a dull boy."

When you work too much and leave no time for your family and personal life, work becomes a burden you feel compelled to bear. This puts you in the pool of stress, and ends up draining your happiness.

To block chronic stress from your life you need find a balance between all of your obligations and needs. Here are a few ways to ensure that:

Try not to bring your work home unless you have a deadline to meet. Make sure you always leave your workplace on time and when you get home, focus only on yourself and your family.

Spend at least an hour or two of quality time with your loved ones daily to keep them and yourself happy.

Devote at least an hour to yourself daily by doing something relaxing.

Build relaxing and soothing rituals that increase your emotional wellbeing. For instance, you could go on a picnic with family every Sunday or watch comedy movies with friends every Saturday. Calming rituals help you take a break from your routine obligations, allowing you to keep stress at bay from yourself.

Get Proper and Sufficient Sleep

All the wear and tear that happens in your body while you are awake gets fixed when you rest. When you sleep, your body relaxes, which helps it overcome the exhaustion it experienced during the day. If you do not sleep well and enough daily, you are likely to become more stressed and irritable.

Research conducted by researchers at the University of Pennsylvania discovered that people who sleep 4.5 hours or less at night are likely to stay more stressed, sad, and angry than those who sleep more. Adults require about 7 to 9 hours of sleep on average and if you are not getting this much sleep, it's no wonder you constantly feel stressed and exhausted.

To ensure you are getting enough sleep, first find out why you are unable to sleep well at night. Is it because you worry too much or because your bed is uncomfortable? Once you know what keeps you from falling asleep easily, look for ways to fix that trouble.

A good exercise is to write down all your worries in a daily in a journal before you go to bed. Tell yourself you will attend to them the next day. Once your worries are out in the open, they stop harassing you and impeding your efforts to sleep.

Switch off your phone and noisy appliances before going to bed and ensure the temperature is comfortable enough to promote a good night's sleep. Do something that is relaxing and soothing an hour before your sleep time so you feel relaxed like take a bath or meditate. It is easier to initiate sleep when you feel relaxed; therefore, unwinding before your sleep time is an extremely effective and important.

Make the above lifestyle changes part of your routine so you can reduce your current stress levels and avoid falling prey to chronic stress. Remind yourself that the right mindset is crucial to avert stress.

Change the Way You Think

Negative thinking does nothing but stress you. Yes, thinking of the worst case scenarios is something you do before embarking on a new journey so you stay prepared for contingencies; however, worrying yourself to death and thinking that only the worst will happen to you is not wise. Studies show that negative thinking is indeed one of the biggest causes of stress, depression, and anxiety. To thwart stress, you have to make changes to your way of thinking.

To develop an attitude that helps you perceive setbacks as learning opportunities, that allows you to see the good in even the worst situations, encourages you to move forward with hope, and to stop attaching negativity to everything that happens against your wishes, you MUST become a positive thinker.

When you develop the ability to think positively, you train your mind to pick out the good things from bad situations. This shifts your focus from upsetting things to more uplifting ones, which helps you become more optimistic in life. In addition, this keeps you from labeling any event as negative or debilitating.

Naturally, when you extract the good from upsetting situations, you perceive everything as an opportunity to grow and become better. This reshapes the way you perceive everything around you, and ensures you never experience chronic stress.

To become a positive thinker, try the following strategies.

Live in the Present

Living in the present and focusing on everything it entails helps you let go of past worries and future concerns. When you dwell in the present, you stop lamenting over what has happened and stop fretting about what may happen. Naturally, when your worries decrease, you find it easy to thwart stress and to think positively.

To do that, do everything mindfully and consciously. If you are doing laundry or writing a book, focus on that task instead of letting your mind wander to something else. Do everything slowly and calmly: become more mindful of it.

As you become more aware of what you are doing, you train your mind to live in the present moment, which consequently diverts your attention away from your worries, thus helping you block stress from your life.

By doing things mindfully, you not only stop living in the past or future, you also increase your involvement in the current task. Naturally, when you become more engaged in a task, you enjoy it more, which causes you to focus on its benefits. This slowly helps you focus on the pros of everything you do thus helping you think positively.

Take Inventory of Your Thoughts

Taking regular inventory of your thoughts is an important part of changing your thought process. If your perception of life is negative, and you nurture a negative attitude, you must take inventory of how you perceive the world in order to change your thought process.

To do that, spend about half an hour with yourself daily. Sit in a quiet room with your journal and think of how you feel about yourself, your life, your accomplishments, and every aspect of your life. If a negative or unhealthy thought pops up, quickly change it to something more optimistic. For instance, if when thinking about your health, you feel, "I am too obese and unattractive," change this thought to, "I am attractive and if I pay more attention to my health, I can look even better." Similarly, if you think, "I know I'll never get the promotion I'm waiting for," change it to "Hard work and smart work can help me get anything even the promotion I'm striving for."

Using this strategy, change all your unhealthy and unconstructive thoughts to uplifting and constructive ones so you push yourself to think along the positive lines. Make a practice out of doing this regularly for at least 20 minutes and you will soon nurture the habit of thinking positively in all circumstances. This practice helps you choose positive thoughts over negative ones, which then help you build an optimistic and healthy mindset because as William James said,

"The greatest weapon against stress is our ability to choose one thought over another."

Practice Incantations

Incantations are positive suggestions you give to yourself to rewire your mind to think a certain way and believe in what you suggest. According to famous self-help guru, Tony Robbins, incantations are arguably one of the best ways to shape a more optimistic mindset and attitude.

Incantations work their magic by encouraging your subconscious to focus on more positive things and suggestions. When your subconscious embraces a positive suggestion, it makes your conscious mind believe in that suggestion, and when you strongly believe in something, you do everything in your power to make it come true.

Your subconscious and conscious minds share a relationship similar to that of the body of the iceberg and its tip. Your conscious mind acts like the tip of the iceberg that is visible to everyone while the subconscious mind behaves like the iceberg's huge lower portion that holds all the power but is invisible to us. Your subconscious mind serves as the driving force behind the conscious mind and influences all the actions taken by your conscious mind.

The subconscious mind is the storage space for everything you learn over the years, all the information you learn, and every memory you form. Your subconscious mind uses this information to influence and direct your conscious mind.

When you behave a certain way and repeat that action over and over again, this thought/behavior creates pathways in your subconscious, and your subconscious mind then directs your conscious mind to behave in that manner each time.

For instance, if you criticize yourself whenever you make mistakes, you are likely to behave that way each time you falter. If you habitually talk to yourself in a negative tone, and see everything under a negative light, it is mainly because you have trained your subconscious mind to think that way.

However, the good news is that you can reprogram your subconscious mind into thinking positively; practicing incantations is an apt way to do so. To exercise this strategy, have a positive suggestion of any change you would like to make in your life— think losing weight, becoming happier, acquiring wealth and abundance or any other positive change you would like to make in your life.

Next, come up with a positive suggestion based on the change you want to make and chant it loudly and clearly. If you want to become positive and happy, you could say, "I am optimistic about life and this makes me happy."

Chant the affirmation with complete belief and visualize what you say. If you are affirming happiness to your subconscious, imagine yourself as the happiest person in the world and smile as you visualize that happy scenario. This increases your involvement in the practice, thus making your brain strengthen the neural pathways conforming to this suggestion. The stronger the neural pathways become, the more firmly the suggestion imbeds into your subconscious.

Practice this exercise for at least 15 minutes daily and within 3 weeks, you will feel more positive and happier than before.

Build a Positive Environment and Support System around You

The people around you directly influence your thoughts and your stress levels. Often, our stress is the result of the venom spewed by the negative people around. Since we fail to recognize those people and understand their poisonous effects on time, we keep letting them wreak havoc in our lives and on our minds.

To avert stress, focus on the sort of people around you most of the time. If you are around naysayers who know nothing else except how to bring you down, these people are responsible for making you feel upset, and you need to dismiss them from your life.

To ensure stress stops lurking in your life, build a healthy, positive environment around you comprising of happy, calm, and optimistic people who encourage you to be better and support you in your decisions. When the right people surround you, you think optimistically and see the good in life.

Take Note of Your Strengths and Blessings

In addition to doing all the above, make a habit of being aware, and appreciative of your strengths and blessings in life. By recognizing your strengths and blessings, you feel good about yourself and your life, which reframes your mind to think positively. This shifts your focus from things you do not have to things you do have resulting in happiness and feelings of calm.

Upon waking up every day, think of 3 personal strengths and 3 blessings in your life. Keep recalling those blessings and strengths the entire day and be grateful for those gifts. For instance, you could acknowledge your compassion, knack for baking, and the loving people in your life that support you through thick and thin.

Write down your strengths and blessings every day and review those entries regularly. This keeps you aware of how blessed you are and helps you block stress before it comes rolling in your life.

These strategies not only help prevent stress, they also help decrease and alleviate your chronic stress. However, other strategies can specifically help you mitigate stress once it affects you. Let us discuss those in the next chapter.

Chapter 9: Breathing Exercises For A Relaxed You

You are suffering from chronic stress, and breathing exercises can be the most important stress-managing tool you can utilize. All the traditional relaxation methods such as meditation and yoga place a central emphasis on breathing.

Deep Breathing Exercise

The practice

Sit comfortably in a chair in a quiet spot in your house. Place one hand just above the belt line and another on your chest. Placing your hands on certain spots will tell you which part of your body and which muscles you are using to breathe.

Slowly open your mouth and sigh. The point of the sigh is to relax the muscles of your upper body. So relax your chest and shoulders.

Gently close your mouth and pause for a few seconds.

Keeping your mouth closed, inhale slowly through your nose. As the air goes in your body, feel your belly rising with the increased pressure of air just under your hand. Continue to breathe in as much air as you can comfortably. Stop when finished inhaling.

Pause for a few moments. Pausing time will be different for different people because every individual and their bodies are different.

Open your mouth and breathe out through our mouth.

Pause.

Repeat the steps 4 to 7.

Often beginners find the practice awkward, especially when first starting out. Don't worry because with practice you will get better at it. See how newborns breathe for real life demonstration.

Alternate Nostril Breathing

Alternate nostril breathing is another effective way to calm your mind when you are feeling stressed.

The practice

Sit comfortably or lie down.

Close your left nostril with the fourth and fifth fingers of your right hand. Then breathe in gently and deeply through your right nostril.

Hold the breath for a few seconds. Then close your right nostril with your thumb. Open your left nostril and breathe out through it.

Repeat the steps two and three for several times

Practice daily

Breathing Retraining

Rapid, shallow breathing also known as hyperventilation can cause symptoms related to stress. Breathing retaining lowers your stress and helps manage symptoms related to stress.

The exercise

Sit or lie on your back in a relaxed spot.

Position your hands on the belly and indicate to your breathing that it shifts toward the center of your body. Notice how your hands start to shift with your belly as you breathe in and breathe out.

Continue to take deep, gentle breaths as you feel more relaxed and comfortable.

Think about an incident or an event that has less importance to you. If you feel any stress, stop thinking about the event and return to abdominal breathing until you start to feel comfortable again.

Then go back to thinking about the event until you can imagine yourself staying calm and relaxed through the whole scenario. Go back to belly breathing anytime you want.

Now choose a situation or an event that has a moderate importance to you. Then repeat the steps 4 and 5.

One by one, move up through difficulty and continue to select situation that results in slightly more anxiety for you. Then repeat steps 4 and 5 until you feel comfortable in each situation.

Chapter 10: How To Reduce Relationship Stress & Family Stress

Do you think the stress meter is going higher in your relationship? In this busy world, you often run after your work and studies, but ignore family and relationship. One of the easiest ways to reduce stress in a relationship is by spending quality time with your partner.

Get closer while facing hardships

Wondering if there are steps you can follow to reduce stress on family and relationship? Well, there are absolutely ways that can help you control stress. Are you looking for ways to help you get closer when such situation arise? Interestingly, hardships really bring you closer to your loved ones. Even though it doesn't mean, they will be immune to stress, working with one another will help you deal with it effectively. All you need is to follow some simple techniques and ways that will help you avoid these stress once and for all. To help you get started, here are some of the ways that you must follow.

Some quick steps to avoid stress in your relationship

Find out the actual cause of stress:

The first step is finding the main cause of stress. Before going deeper with the situation, you need to first find the root cause of stress. If you are feeling stress in your relationship, find out what is causing it. This means, find out if the cause is external or within the relationship. If the source is external, don't try to deal with it as a relationship problem. Often, money can become a relationship problem, but in reality money is a fiscal problem. It becomes a relationship issue if you allow it. The best way is working as a team and solving relationship issues.

Stop making negative assumptions about any situation:

If something happens where you don't have control, never make the situation worse by making assumptions. For instance, if someone loses their job, you don't need to mention they will also lose their home. However, instead of the negative assumptions, simply talk to your partner or family member and try to bring up a solution. Above all, never let stress win over the situation since it is the time to show your loved ones that you care.

Don't blame or be too critical:

After you find out about a situation in your family or your spouse's life, never start with the blame game. This is one of the factors that results in the destruction of peace in the family and contributes to stress. Your main aim should be to move closer to your partner. The same applies for being extremely critical. Face the fact that sometimes things go wrong and there is nothing you can do about it. Look at every challenge as a means to strengthen the bond between the both of you. This will help you reduce stress and avoid the blame game.

Take one day off from work and spend time with your spouse:

Your partner needs you in her crisis. So, it is important to make your presence felt. Try to take a day off from your busy schedule and spend time with her. Reassure her that you are always there for her no matter goes wrong. This will helps prevent relationship stress and bring you closer. It is always a great idea to let your partner know how important she is in your life. There is no better way to prove it than by spending one whole day with her.

Acknowledge your spouse's concern:

When something goes wrong and you are responsible for that, there are chances for you to turn defensive, especially when your spouse or partner shows concern. What you need to do is stop confrontation with your partner by putting away your ego. You need to acknowledge their concern with all your heart. This really helps in avoiding family and relationship stress. You need to make yourself understand that since you both are partners, you both are in this situation, together. So, it is perfectly fine that you have similar concerns and the best way is to cooperate with one another.

Don't react, but respond:

Reacting too quickly is one of the things you better avoid if you want to avoid stress. Instead, bring on the habit of responding. For instance, when you react to a bad news, it is normal that you will give negative comments. If you respond, your knee jerking reaction will be in control and so you will be able to deal with the situation. Without doubt, response helps you avoid stress as well as allow you to make room for positive emotions such as understanding and compassion.

Respect each other's feelings:

The next most important thing is to respect each other as well as your feelings. Usually, the way women and men react to stress is quite different. The man might think that the women is attaching excessive emotion to the situation, which isn't necessary. Again, the woman might feel that the man is ignoring the problem and the situation. Just by understanding the fact they both men and women respond to stress differently help you deal with the situation well.

Look out for opportunities to help one another:

How does it feel when your spouse has confidence in you? It is a great feeling isn't it. Well, it is really true, especially during the difficult times when you don't yourself. There is simply nothing that gives you confidence and lifts you up like the confidence of your loved ones. Due to this, mutual encouragement is the primary factor to reduce stress. Rather than waiting for stressful situations to arrive, it is better to make the most of every opportunity to be one another.

With that being said, you need to know that stressful situations can arrive anytime without knocking at your door. You need to be prepared to face anything that comes your way be. By following these steps you can easily reduce and avoid relationship and family stress every time. Lastly, remember every solution starts with you. So, you need to have faith in yourself and your family to be able to overcome it.

Chapter 11: Quick Fixes To Turn Your Day Around

Stressful situations can come on any typical day. Even if you're just spending most of your time at home or most especially in the office, stressors are always present. Stress is also experienced by anyone no matter what age, gender, or race. What matters is how you deal with it.

One of my favorite quotes goes: "Life's energy is what you make it. Make it purposeful, positive, fulfilling, and great." However, how can you make things great if things are so stressful? Here are some quick fixes to reduce or eliminate stress:

Take Deep Breaths

Don't underestimate the power of taking deep breaths whenever you're stressed or overwhelmed with emotions. According to research, breathing exercises help increase the flow of oxygen to the brain; regulate the blood pressure, and lower cortisol levels, which could help reduce stress and anxiety.

Do the following steps the next time you're faced with a stressful situation: 1. Pull your back up and sit straight. If possible, you could also try lying on the floor. 2. Inhale, taking in as much air as you can through your nose (your stomach should be rising when you're inhaling). 3. Exhale slowly through your mouth (you must feel your abdominal muscles contracting). 4. Do this repeatedly until you feel the stress in your body reducing.

Relax Your Muscles

Do you feel tired both physically and mentally? Release that tension in your body first! One relaxation technique you can use as a quick fix for stress is what is known as "progressive relaxation." This refers to a therapy that involves tensing and relaxing the muscles in your body one at a time. Hold one muscle group in your body (for example, your shoulders) for a few seconds and then carefully relax them to release the tension. You can start with your shoulders, then your arms, your abdomen, etc. Once your body is free from stress, you will notice that you are also releasing stress mentally.

Get a Time Out

If you feel that the situation is just too much, it would be best if you give yourself a break. Go to a place or find a corner that will help you release stress and feel relaxed. One thing that you can do is to take a quick stroll outside; you'll see that walking at least one block could help reduce your stress. In fact, research shows that walking helps increase the flow of oxygen in the body and increases the production of hormones called endorphins that help calm you down.

Talk to Someone

Sometimes, talking about why you're stressed to a person you trust is all it takes for you to calm down. Venting your feelings to a person who supports you might not only help release stress, but that individual could also help talk some sense into you by giving you a different perspective.

Release Stress through Writing

Again, keeping a journal really helps a lot with managing your stress level. This could mean a little effort (because you have to write everything down: how you felt, how you dealt with the situation, etc.), but you might find this very therapeutic, especially if you're looking for a fast way to control your stress.

Listen to Music

This is another easy way to release stress in your body. According to research, listening to classical music, such as Pachelbel's Canon could help control anxiety, manage hypertension, and lower heart rates. Another study showed that listening to music is also beneficial to cancer patients who are undergoing chemotherapy. The research reported that patients who listened to music during their treatment showed good mood, controlled blood pressure, and lower heart rate.

Try Laughing

Whenever you feel that the things happening at your office are just too much, why don't you take a break by watching your favorite stand-up comedian on YouTube? According to experts, laughing, whether it's just a giggle or loud chuckling, is proven to reduce stress. Scientists found that laughter increases the flow of oxygen, which helps the body release tension that is caused by stress.

Can't laugh? Even a forced smile could change your mood! Research has shown that a smile, even if it's not based on real emotion, can elevate one's mood.

Have Tea

One research in the UK found that drinking tea could improve someone's mood and reduce the effects of stress and anxiety. The study involved two groups, which took tests to measure their anxiety levels. After that, they were instructed to take on a stress-inducing task, which they had to finish in a certain amount of time. After the test, the first group was asked to drink a cup of tea, while the second group drank only water, and both groups were asked again to take a test that would measure their anxiety. The result of the experiment showed that the groups had significant differences in terms of their stress levels. The group that drank water had an average 25% increase of anxiety after the task; while the first group who drank tea had a 4% drop in their anxiety levels. Scientists who administered the test explain that most people associate drinking tea with relaxation, which helps trigger the brain to recover from stress. Next time you're stressed, remember to get a quick fix by drinking a hot cup of old-fashioned black tea.

Get a Massage

Whether it's shiatsu, Swedish, or a traditional Thai massage, research shows that massage therapy does not only help reduce physical pain, but is also an effective way to fight stress. One research study noted the participants in the experiment had lower levels of cortisol (a stress hormone) in their saliva after they were massaged. Other studies showed that massage therapy can release muscle tension, improve mood, and promote quality of sleep.

Light Aromatic Candles or Oils

For thousands of years, aromatherapy has been used to address a variety of ailments using different kinds of scents. Today, aromatherapy is also used as a holistic treatment to beat symptoms of stress like pain and fatigue. Lighting aromatic oils or candles (like lavender, lemon, and linaloe wood) in your home or in your workstation has been proven to create a relaxing environment that can lift your mood and diminish stress.

Use Art as Therapy

Do you enjoy sketching or painting? How about scrapbooking? Why don't you use your love for the arts as your outlet to relieve stress? In fact, many studies in the past have shown that using art as therapy is an effective way to manage stress.

Kiss or Hug Your Loved One

Had a tiring day at work? One way to release stress before turning in for the day is to show affection to your kids, spouse, or loved one by kissing or hugging them.

According to research, kissing triggers the brain to release chemicals such as serotonin, oxytocin, and dopamine that are also known as "feel-good hormones." Like kissing, hugging can lower blood pressure and stress levels.

Chapter 12: Handling And Management Of Stress

How do we manage stress? How do we cope up with difficulties and how do we turn our self to a medical solution without creating an additional string of stress? Isn't it likewise stressful to accept the fact that we need medical attention because our system failed to handle stress? There could be a hundred ways to handle stress from simple time management up to seeking medical attention. Crossing our path every day with a different kind of stressor is comparable to a game, and like any game, there is a winner and a loser. Choosing who will win mirror the way individual handle stress.

Before birth, the responsibility to handle stress rests on the mother. Seeing a pregnant woman smoking because she feels relieved through smoking cure her emotional stressor and of a child to some extent but not the health stressor, the effect of smoking to a child. The best way to handle stress for babies inside the womb is to address the stressor of a mother. Each stage of life has its unique way of handling or managing stress but in general, the most common are the following:

Immediate Family and Friends. There should be an acceptance that we are just human being and we alone cannot handle everything. Life is simply like that. It is not a fairy tale to live but a continuous struggle to survive. Remember the notion that no man is an island; we need to find strength in another person. The same reason why the term friends are invented anyway, they are that person whom we can turn to in cases of joy and in the struggle.

A child does not have the ability to accept things or difficulties in life but through parents, anything will be managed, and a child will be able to understand. During a stressful time, a teenager will not seek the help of a mother but of immediate friends. Because the adult's ego dictates otherwise most of the times, they need friends and a partner who can direct them realities of life.

Medical Help. Stressor attack our body system makes them weak and susceptible to disease. This is where the role of medicine and science in handling and managing stress is badly needed. The effect of chronic stress requires medical attention, simply because your body can no longer handle it nor alternative medicine. Do not hesitate to consult experts and medical practitioners depending on your need. Chronic stress requires science and human expertise to mitigate. Depression is real and can lead to death if not mitigated. While we have friends and family and they are our immediate relief to depression, but the thing is stress attacks when a person is alone.

The first strike of stress is in your central nervous system, the one that directs your brain and your command of your body. The excessive function of your nervous system is dangerous, your heartbeat will continue to pump and so with your body organs. You can experience frequent urination, vomiting, headaches and muscle pain among others. Stress can also lower your immune system which can lead to infections and weaken the antibodies against other infectious diseases. Accept the fact that there are things in life that only science can answer, chronic stress needs that.

Finding Inner Strength – Our body has healing capacity. Look at how the wounds heal on its own. We have antibodies that shield our body from harmful intruders. Antibodies are also known as immunoglobulins produced by our immune system to help stop viruses, bacteria, or other chemicals from harming the body. Hence, we can fight stress from within.

Psychologically, inner strength is the one that keeps you moving and cause you to live. It makes you happy, makes you at peace and produces that feeling of safety and security. It can come from within and reinforced by our attachment. It supposed to answer the questions of what makes you happy and contended. You can look at your activities like swimming, dancing, singing, gardening, and cooking. Activities that detach you from the stress and instead makes you at peace. Most women see shopping and a massage an effective stress reliever. This is also where enriching your passion starts, finding where you are good at, finding your music and exploring arts.

Inner strength can also be reinforced by investing in conversing with your trusted friends and being with someone who could make you feels safe. Finding inner strength can help you address the harmful effect of stress in your body. While being passive sometimes is helpful, so that you will not be affected, but it should not be practiced all the times.

Seek Nature's Help. This is seeing the beauty of nature to feel relieved and has that sense of happiness. Corny as it can be but seeing a beautiful flower can make an individual smile. Every time a smile crosses your face, a party is happening in your brain. It will release hormones called endorphins which can calm your nervous system. A relax nervous system allows your body to function well, it can lower heart rate and blood pressure.

The wonder of nature also includes any creature living with it including humans. But let's deal more on the goodness of having pets around even if your pet is a snake. You can talk to them and they will listen, just do not expect them to talk back. If you do, that is a sign that you need medical attention. Pets can make you happy and can comfort you.

Strengthening Faith. This is about using your belief and religion to address and mitigate the effect of stress. Live with your faith whatever your religion is, sing their song and listen to the teaching. The true essence of curing a disease goes beyond the healing of the physical body but of mind and soul. Stress can magnify or accelerate a particular medical condition but capitalizing on our faith can be of help. A person just needs to believe.

Stress is a disease and it can be fatal. The irony of a disease is that it can enter our body like a flash of light, but it takes time and patience to arrest it.

Handling and Management of Stress

We crossed our path every day with different kinds of stressor, and as a game there is a winner and a loser. Choosing who will win mirror the way an individual handle and manage stress.

Life is simply like that. It is not a fairy tale to live but a continuous struggle to survive. We sometimes cannot do it alone; we need to find strength in another person. The same reason why the term friends are invented.

Inner strength is the one that keeps you moving and cause you to live. It makes you happy, makes you at peace and produces that feeling of safety and security.

Corny as it can be but seeing a beautiful flower can make an individual smile. Every time a smile crosses your face, a party is happening in your brain. It will release hormones called endorphins which can calm your nervous system. A relax nervous system allows your body to function well, it can lower heart rate and blood pressure.

Live with your faith whatever your religion is, sing their song and listen to the teaching. The true essence of curing a disease goes beyond the healing of the physical body but of mind and soul.

Chapter 13: Lifestyle Habits Which Relieve Stress

So, smoking, drinking too much, not getting enough sleep, overdosing on caffeine and hanging around people who stress you out can all contribute to your stress levels rising through the roof. But, when you try to give up these harmful habits in order to help with your stress and anxiety, which ones are the best to replace them with? Often, replacing a habit with another habit can be a great way to help you quit the first one. For example, those who smoke may want to replace smoking cigarettes with vaping, which is less harmful but provides them with something to do instead of lighting up a cigarette. Others prefer to swap harmful habits for good habits which are drastically different – for example, someone who drinks too much alcohol may decide to start lifting weights to give them something else to do instead of having a drink.

Exercise

We've dedicated a whole chapter of this book to exercise already, but it's so important that it needed to be mentioned again. Regular exercise is one of the best lifestyle habits that you can have when it comes to improving your mental health and making sure that your stress levels are under control. Taking part in activities such as walking, running, cycling, swimming, yoga, and even weight lifting or playing a team sport can boost physical fitness, improve strength, and increase self-esteem and confidence, all of which can help to improve stress and anxiety. Exercising itself releases feel-good chemicals in the brain, and has been clinically proven to reduce the symptoms of anxiety and depression.

Meditation

When it comes to combatting stress, meditation is a great habit to take up and integrate into your lifestyle. For centuries, meditation has been used to help people deal with their stress and anxiety levels and feel calmer within themselves. Meditation helps you to find the positive energy inside of yourself and feel more connected and at peace with yourself and the world around you. Those who meditate regularly find that stressful situations no longer overwhelm them as much; they are calmer, more relaxed, and able to take on more and more. Whether you are a spiritual person or not, there is no doubt that mindfulness meditation can help you to feel more relaxed and in control. Even the act of taking the time to sit in quiet and collect your thoughts for a while can help to reduce stress, as meditation requires you to breathe deeply, which will oxygenate your brain and give you more energy to deal with your stress. Mindfulness mediation can be done at home, or in a class. You can also use a range of essential oils or music to aid you.

Creativity

Getting creative can be one of the best ways to deal with stress. And, the best thing about using creativity to combat stress is that you don't have to be particularly artistic in order to so successfully. There have been many studies which directly relate getting creative to lower stress levels, with adult coloring books and apps for stress being a huge success. The simple act of coloring in pictures, or perhaps doing something creative such as baking, needlework or even DIY, can be very therapeutic and can distract your thoughts and focus from your stress and on to something else. So, if you're feeling stressed out, it might be time to think about taking up a new creative hobby.

Friends and Family

People who are mentally strong do not dissociate themselves from those who are closest to them. When you're feeling stressed out, it can be easy to try and hide your stress levels from your family members and close friends as naturally, you don't want them to be worried about you. However, knowing when to ask for support and having the best people around you to offer that can be very important when it comes to effectively managing stress. Building and maintaining strong relationships with your family and close friends means that you will have somebody to talk to when the going gets tough, which can be extremely helpful for stress. Having somebody to talk to and confide in about whatever is stressing you out can help you by giving you an outsider's perspective, which can often help by putting your own thoughts into a better perspective. Along with that, having people to turn to can stop you from taking too much on yourself, giving you more time to relax and keep on top of your mental health.

Chapter 14: Identifying Disorders Caused By Stress

When coping with high levels of stress over an extended period of time, it is more than likely that a person will develop a mental or physical disorder. Some of these afflictions are not so serious, while others can be life threatening. When ignored or left untreated, these conditions can become very serious. People often ignore stress-caused illnesses because they believe the condition will pass, or that their stress is only temporary. Unfortunately, this is false.

We will first discuss minor, more common afflictions caused by stress. One of the most common stress related problems are headaches. What exactly is a headache? A headache is pain or distress in the head. While there are countless reasons that headaches occur, stress is one of the major factors. Some people experience chronic, constant headaches, while others only get them occasionally.

There are two major types of headaches, primary and secondary. It is important to identify which one you have. In the category of primary headaches, tension, migraine, and cluster headaches are included. Tension headaches are minor, everyday headaches, mainly caused by high levels of stress. Migraine headaches are slightly worse, and affect women more than men. They can cause a great deal of pain, and a complete inability to focus. Cluster headaches are a very rare type of headache. They are repeated and painful, and those afflicted suffer every day. In many cases, secondary types of medicine are resorted to treat these serious headaches. Fortunately, cluster headaches rarely occur.

How can we manage primary headaches? Medications such as Advil are the most popular treatments. For the large majority of people, headaches are an annoyance, but not a health risk. To reduce the frequency and intensity of your headaches, meditate, and use the stress reduction techniques discussed in this book! The chances of getting a headache reduce tremendously if you are feeling calm and relaxed throughout your day. As you become better at managing stress, you should notice a definite improvement in your ability to control annoyances such as headaches.

The next categories we will discuss are secondary headaches. For the large part, secondary headaches are more serious than primary headaches. Secondary headaches stem from physical injuries or conditions. Concussive and traumatic headaches fall into this category. There is not nearly as much research done on secondary headaches as primary. This is due to the fact that secondary headaches are set offs from a more major problem in the body. It is assumed that these types of headaches are caused by these injuries or afflictions, but we cannot be sure at this point. If you believe you are experiencing secondary headaches, the best thing to do is go to a medical doctor and be checked out.

Depression/anxiety are also afflictions caused by stress. Depression is a medical condition, which results in constant sadness/numbness, feelings of worthlessness, among many other symptoms. When constantly bombarded by stress without correctly managing it, the brain does not react very well at all. A common reaction to being overly stressed out is to simply "give up." "Giving up" leads to loss of interest in hobbies, losing contact with friends, and ultimately transforms into full-scale depression. Anxiety is slightly different than depression, with symptoms including nervousness, paranoia, and uneasiness.

When under a heavy stress load, some people instead of becoming sad or giving up, do the opposite. Questions begin to pop up in their minds like "What if I can't do this?" "There is no way I can get that done" or "My boss is definitely out to get me." For our purposes, know that anxiety, in this case caused by stress, is a coping mechanism. People will try to affirm to themselves that there is no way they can deal with what is going on in their lives simply because they believe they are unable to. Feelings of people being out to get you and uneasiness in social situations are also common. We can help get rid of anxiety by using our stress reduction techniques, while also using the following method.

If you know you have stress related anxiety, there is fortunately a few ways that we can deal with it and help cure it. Unlike depression, which can be more detrimental and long lasting, anxiety is a disorder that is more easily treated. The first step is acknowledging that you have anxiety. Many people nervously believe that there is no way they have such a condition, and that the people who tell them they do are simply crazy and do not know what they are talking about.

The first method to combat your anxiety is writing down reasons you feel causes it.

Make a list of all the things that make you anxious. Read them out loud, and you will begin to rule out the reasons that seem ridiculous or unreasonable. For example, you might write down that you fear you will get arrested for drunk driving. However, if you fear it that much, it is very doubtful that you will even put yourself in the situation in which you can get arrested for drunk driving. After you rule out the unreasonable reasons, there will be handfuls that are legitimate. Maybe you are anxious because you believe your boss is going to fire you, or that your car will break down on the way to work. Instead of ignoring and living with these insecurities, the best way to knock them down is to confront them directly.

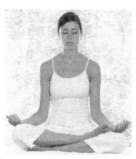

Managers also have a large part in reducing workplace stress. Man

Let's say you identified the fear of being fired as a reason for your anxiety. How do we confront this fear? Well, first take the steps that are directly in your control. How does a good employee behave? Showing up early to work, completing all tasks in a timely manner, and not just being at work, but also being at work to help others get better at what they do. Make a conscious effort to give your boss a reason to promote you, not fire you. What we just did was reverse your psychology. Instead of living with the fear of being fired, live with the fire under you that you must do everything in your power to earn a promotion.

How about another example? As said before, let's say that one of the causes of your stress-induced anxiety is that you fear your car will break down on the way to work or an important event. Instead of fearing your car will break down, do everything in your power to prevent that from happening. Use better gas, get an oil change, and get new tires, anything to affirm to you that the car is in too good of a shape to break down. Irrationalize your fears. Try to do so much to prevent unlikely bad events from occurring that you remove even the slightest glimmer in your mind that anything unfortunate will happen.

Now, of course, not everything will go perfectly in your life. Like with all people, things will go wrong. But when they do, do not let anxiety take over. Realize that bad events happen to all people, and now that it happened, you will do everything in your power to prevent it from happening again. When combating anxiety, acknowledge that attitude and mentality are everything.

Chapter 15: Aromatherapy

Aromatherapy entails the use of scent to transform the way you feel. When you inhale air, which is infused with essential oils, it usually goes to the roof of your nose where the olfactory receptors within the nose transport this information to the limbic system (where emotions are usually processed). This in turn triggers the release of feel good chemicals that enable the brain to relax.

Some of the common essential oils that you can use for this purpose include:

Sandalwood essential oil

Peppermint essential oil

German chamomile essential oil

Lavender essential oil

Almond essential oil

Eucalyptus essential oil

Clary sage essential oil (this one helps with sleep)

How to use the essential oils:

-Apply a few drops onto your hands and then breathe deeply.

-Apply a few drops onto your chest and then try breathing in the aroma

-Apply the oils to your handkerchief, clothes or pillow or other stuff you can easily or regularly inhale

-Apply a few drops (one or two) on the crown of your head or along the back of the neck then breath in with a bottle of the essential oil right under the nose.

Note: Only get natural or unprocessed oils free from additives. Read the labels well to ensure that you obtain proper oils. Also, ensure to dilute essential oils with carrier oils for safety.

Decompress

To relax your muscles and calm the mind, place a warm heat wrap around the neck and shoulders for around 10 minutes. Close your eyes and then relax the face, neck, back muscles and the chest. Then remove the heat wrap and now use a foam roller or tennis ball to massage the tension away.

-Put the ball between the wall and your back.

-Lean into the ball, and then hold gentle pressure for about 10-20 seconds

-Now move the ball to a different spot and apply pressure in a similar manner

Create a Morning Ritual

What you do in the morning greatly determines how your day will be. So if you start badly, your day will be a reflection of just that. The truth is that you cannot be rolling out of bed with your smartphone tightly held on your hands to check the latest social media updates. If the first thing that you hear is the annoying alarm, this simply means that you start your day subconsciously "stressed". You also will end up stressed throughout the day if the first thing you see in the morning is news of how the world's economy is doing bad, how people are dying and lots of other things. And if you see updates from your friends sharing their good times, you end up feeling bad about yourself (let's be honest, you feel sort of jealous and as if you are missing out). You need to change your morning ritual to include things that help you stay grounded and connected to your present moment.

When you wake up, the first thing you need to do is to just be with yourself. Reflect on your life, count your blessings, thank the universe for a good day ahead, light a candle, or burn incense, meditate etc. Just ensure to do something that keeps you truly grounded in your present and forget about the technology and stresses of the world. Anything that helps you to focus on yourself and not your to do list is good enough for you. Savor every moment in the morning and strive to nurture a habit of doing just that every morning. Here is a sample morning ritual:

Wake up at 5am

Freshen up and say a prayer

Head for the morning run at 5.15am-5.30am

Meditate for 10 minutes or do a deep breathing exercise from 5.30am-5.40am

Shower as you prepare breakfast 5.45am-6am

Breakfast 6am-6.20am

Prepare your to dos for the day 6.20am-6.30am

Head to work 6.45am

You can tweak the morning ritual to suit your lifestyle. As you saw from the above sample morning ritual, I didn't talk about calling a friend, checking the latest tweets, updating your Facebook profile, catching up with the latest news etc. Your goal is to center on yourself every morning and just live as if nothing else matters to you. In doing that, you will ultimately find yourself happier and less stressed. As I said, how your day starts determines how it will progress.

Eat It

What you eat has a profound effect on your ability to deal with stressful situations in life. Actually, some foods might even be the ones that contribute to stress in your life. Although this doesn't mean that you should avoid them, it is important to take them in moderation. Some of the foods that might aggravate stress include alcohol, soda (soft drinks), tea, fast foods, sugar etc. So what foods should you be eating?

Chapter 16: Rain

Meditation teacher and psychologist Tara Brach described RAIN as a four-step process that can help you deal with stress and difficult situations better. It stands for:

R – recognizing what is happening;

A – allowing life to be just as it is;

I – investigating inner experience with kindness; and

N – non-identification or realizing that people are not limited or defined by their emotions.

Steps on How to Practice RAIN

First of all, you need to recognize any strong emotions that you may be feeling. Stop whatever you are doing and focus on this emotion. Once you recognize it, you should gently move away from it. Observe it in a non-judgmental manner instead.

Stay present in the moment. You can also label your feelings. For instance, you may say that you are feeling overwhelmed or stressed. When you recognize how you feel, you can open up an inner space and bring you into contact with yourself and the present moment.

Next, you need to allow or simply let it be. You have to acknowledge and accept the reality of your present moment. You do not have to like or love the situation. You just have to accept it. Let go of any mental resistance.

Oftentimes, people have an unconscious impulse to suppress, ignore, or push away strong emotions. If you have an internal struggle, you will experience more tension and stress. You will be caught up in your emotions and thoughts before you can even react towards them.

So, you have to allow yourself to experience the present moment. Do not resist it. Be open to it, and you will feel a sense of ease and relaxation.

Once you have recognized and allowed your emotion to exist, you have to investigate it. Ask yourself questions such as why you feel that way or if there are any events that may have influenced such emotion. Determine any factor that may have something to do with it.

Find logical answers to your questions. These answers will help you determine your next course of actions. Through investigation, you will be able to respond properly. It will help you dissolve or resolve your strong emotions so that they will not overcome you.

Finally, you have to practice non-identification. You have to realize that your feelings and thoughts do not define you. Keep in mind that there is always a reason behind every sense perception, thought, and emotion that you have.

When you realize this fact, you will have a sense of ease and freedom. You will have peace of mind. Your emotions and thoughts will not overcome you, no matter how painful or intense they are.

The RAIN technique is simple yet powerful. It is ideal to practice it every time you are faced with a difficult or challenging situation and you need to clear your mind right away. Remember that you have to deal with your situation as soon as possible so that you can prevent saying or doing anything that you might regret later. Stressful situations can bring about unpleasant consequences. Hence, you should know how to deal with them properly.

Chapter 17: Work Ethic

"The only place success comes before work is in the dictionary." Vince Lombardi

Of all the steps toward success this is probably the one we least want to hear about and yet, when questioned on the subject, every successful person, be they a billionaire businessman or a ballet dancer, will tell of the work they had to put in in order to achieve that success. For many of us our minds shy from the thought of grueling hours doing unpleasant and un-stimulating tasks. We like to imagine successful people as those with huge amounts of talent and a natural gift that took them toward their achievement. Research reveals that this is often far from the truth. Many top executives do not have outstanding qualifications or unlimited intellect. The one thing they do have is a huge capacity to work hard.

To look at how they manage to do this we need to go back to that initial vision we talked about in the chapter on passion. Though these people put in long hours at the office or in training those hours are not the painful grind that we might imagine them to be. Many of them suggest that those work hours are some of the most stimulating and positive hours of their day. They do not become successful through plugging away at something they hate doing. Instead they choose to do what they do and it is this reason that makes discovering your passion so crucial to success. Without it you may still succeed in the accepted definition of success that this world so readily adheres to, but you will lack the genuine self-fulfillment that is part of true success.

If we look at work from the perspective of doing something we are passionate about and enjoy doing, then it becomes a little harder to define than what we might normally think of. Many artists and composers talk of becoming so involved in their project that they almost lose sense of time passing. The task ceases to be work and instead transforms into the pursuit of a goal. For real success to be achieved the rewards need to be more holistic than simply the attainment of an end goal. Instead the goal is just part of an overall package.

While it is important to realize that success without work is impossible, work is somehow transformed by passion. At the same time, one should not underestimate the effort that success requires. There are going to be many times that you need to dig deep to keep going. Those successful role models you have do not come home after a sixteen-hour day jumping in the air and kicking their heels together. They will be tired. The difference between them and the guy who has just busted his gut doing a job he hates is that they have a deep sense of self-satisfaction. That world famous golfer who seems to drive a ball so effortlessly toward the green will no doubt tell you of all the work he put in in order to play his game so well. He may have spent hour after hour practicing and had to overcome many motivational setbacks to keep going, but at the end of the day he did all that because he had harnessed his passion.

Research shows that many people are actually happier when they work than when they relax. We may think we would be happier lying sprawled on the couch watching daytime television but work can create many rewards. It provides a sense of achievement, encourages social cohesion and gives our lives a sense of purpose; doing nothing, on the other hand, can develop into a state of apathy that, in extreme cases, may lead to deep depression. Hard work creates value and an inner sense of self-worth that is one reason that the long-term unemployed are so much more vulnerable to mental illness than other sectors of society.

For the individual striving for success the rewards of hard work may be even greater than those of the average working man or woman. Though he still may need to develop discipline and habits to do the hard work he has the advantage of a vision and goal that many people are not so lucky to have. However, you cut it, hard work and success go hand in hand. Passion and a vision are what differentiate between those working toward success and those just doing a job to put bread on the table.

Work ethic is not something that everyone possesses but that does not mean it is beyond their reach.

There are 3 characteristics that define good work ethic:

● Dedication - people with good work ethic work hard at what they do and will do anything to achieve their goals and to ensure they are performing to the best of their abilities at all times.

● Productivity - people with good work ethics are usually highly productive in the work place and will use their time wisely. Being lazy is not in their nature.

● Reliability - people with good work ethics deliver on what they have promised and value punctuality. Deadlines are met and quality is never compromised.

Work ethics need to be applied to every decision you make regarding work or situations in the work place. Making unethical decisions or reacting unethically in certain situations could result is your employees losing interest and focus on their work and affect productivity and delays in your project. You should always think you yourself what would happen should everyone react in the same way you did to a situation, what would the outcome be? Lead by example, you staff follow you lead and if you work ethic is good you will rub off on to them.

Punctuality is a work ethic that cannot be ignored. If you are late for a meeting it shows complete and utter disregard for the person with which you are meeting. It may lead them to think you disrespect them or that you feel their time is not as valuable as yours. This is not a good footing on which to start a prospective business association. Lack of punctuality may also relay the thought that if you can't make a simple meeting on time, how on Earth will you cope with submitting projects on time and under stressful situations. Not being punctual really does nothing to boost confidence in you at all.

Ethics is basically knowing the difference between right and wrong and acting accordingly. Personal ethics will usually stem from your upbringing and experiences while work ethic or professional ethics may stem from your education, and also by the codes of conduct expected in your profession.

If you want people to support your ideas, they need to trust you. Good work ethics will ensure that people see you as the one to trust when things need to be done on time and in the correct manner. People are more likely to cooperate with you if they trust you and value your opinion.

Taking pride in everything you do is great work ethics. From your appearance to your presentations. Give excellent first impressions always and show you work ethics from the start. Arrive on time and dress professionally. The person you are meeting certainly warrants that attention to detail as they have taken the time out of their schedule to meet with you regarding your project. They value the success of your project and want to help you succeed but of course you need to show that you want that too. Take pride in work you present or submit. If something is not done to your standards, don't submit it, rather ask for a small extension with a valid explanation. The client will certainly value your honesty, integrity and the fact that you don't want to submit substandard work as this is a reflection on your capabilities and work ethics. Never go into a meeting unprepared. If your project is that important to you, you will want to showcase your attention to detail and the pride you take in your work. Who would you prefer to take on your project? A sloppy, late, unprepared person or the one who has all his ducks in a row? And

153

honestly which person do you want to portray?

Honesty and transparency are great work ethics to have as part of your arsenal. If you are open and transparent about your project, the successes to date as well as the setbacks and how you have overcome them, people will be more willing to trust your opinions and value your input. Being deceitful and hiding your misgivings is a sure way to disaster. Not everybody can be perfect all the time and to try to portray that you are is surely not believable to begin with. As the saying goes "if it seems too good to be true, it usually is." Be honest and upfront and you will be respected for that.

Being cooperative and a willingness to cooperate in a team environment is an excellent value to have as part of your work ethics. People with good work ethics will value and appreciate the effectiveness of cooperation in getting the tasks completed successfully and efficiently. A person with good work ethics will work in cooperation with whoever is necessary in order to get the project to success. Personal issues are put aside for the sake of the project at hand.

A strong character is usually a trait that people with strong work ethic have at their disposal. Strong character allows them to be self-driven with a willingness to push themselves to the limits to complete the task at hand without having to rely on others or have others intervene.

All the traits discussed which pertain to work ethic are important in allowing others to view you as a person on their way to success and happiness with no fear of the unknown.

Fear of the unknown, fear of failure, fear of eventually giving up are all very real and reasons why some people just don't bother with starting in the first place. They are simply not prepared or mentally strong enough to take failures, setbacks or obstacles in their stride and to see them as learning possibilities. That is exactly what they are, learning possibilities. You learn how to react or diffuse that particular situation in the future so that it is no longer a threat. You learn about yourself and about strengths that you never knew you possessed and would never have known if you didn't take the risk on your dream. You learn whether you dream truly is what you are passionate about. You learn so much about the people who you trust. You learn whether they truly are there for you through thick and thin or whether they are only along for the joy ride. You learn to accept and acknowledge that you don't know everything and too willing seek advice from those who know more in particular areas. The road to success is not a time to worry about what others will think if you ask for advice or help in a particular situation. Rome wasn't built in a day and certainly not by one person on his own.

In order to reach success, you need to possess skills within yourself but do not be led to believe that arrogance and thinking you can do it all alone are going to get you there any faster. Be prepared to accept help where necessary and to give out recognition where it is warranted. Treat others with respect and professionalism and you will draw that attention back to yourself. If you are aware that certain aspects are not your strong point, employ the help of someone who is strong in those points. At the end of your project is your dream and you should want the best possible result to be the outcome. The outcome is a reflection of who you are, what your beliefs are and it allows others to realize your dream in its full glory. You should want this and should employ whatever measures necessary to get there.

A project takes trained hands too complete successfully. The vision is yours but it may take a team to complete it successfully and to your satisfaction. Ensure that you have people around you that are trust worthy and have your best interest at heart and the desire for you to succeed. Your contacts can make or break you so be careful in whom you lay your trust.

At the end of the day, your success and your happiness are in your own hands. The thoughts and mental vibes you put out are what you will receive back. If you really want something you need to make a decision to go out and get it at any cost. See your success in your mind's eye and revel in the pride and fulfillment and this alone should give you the will to physically succeed. Don't leave the possibility of your success in the hand of another, take control and show strong character in the face of adversity. Succeeding against all odds will offer you a feeling of pure satisfaction and guess what, your self-confidence and belief in your abilities will grow tenfold. Bigger and better projects on your horizon and you definitely know you have what it takes to succeed.

Quitters will never experience the joy and elation of success to the fullest. They will never know the feeling of overcoming obstacles and they will never know the true happiness of succeeding and realizing their full potential. Quitters are often people of negative thoughts and mindset who have given up before they even begin. Always be positive and happy with whatever you choose to do and you are half way to success already.

Sometimes in life you have to take risks to get the desired results. When you decide on the risk you are willing to take, dive in head first and don't look back. Don't leave room for what if's or I should have's. Get the job done. Take the plunge and follow your dreams, regret is something that will kill your soul and set you on a downward spiral. What you must realize is each small victory is a step closer to success. If a task seems too large to take on at once, break it up into phases and tackle these one at a time. This will seem more manageable and as you progress through the phases successfully it will boost your confidence and joy through the following phases.

There are really so many ways to go about successfully completing a project and following your passion. How you go about it is entirely up to you. Perhaps you are someone who thrives taking on large projects or maybe you need smaller projects. Plan accordingly but never give up. If you get knocked down, get back up again and come out fighting. This is a winning attitude.

We all have the potential to be winners, successful and happy. Master the skills required with practice, practice and more practice. It will be worth it in the end.

Chapter 18: Stress In The Workplace

Managing Job and Work Stress

While some workplace stress is normal, excessive stress can interfere with your productivity and performance, impact your physical and emotional health, and affect your relationships and home life. It can even determine success or failure on the job. You can't control everything in your work environment, but that doesn't mean you're powerless, even when you're stuck in a difficult situation. Whatever your ambitions or work demands, there are steps you can take to protect yourself from the damaging effects of stress, improve your job satisfaction, and bolster your well-being in and out of the workplace.

When Is Workplace Stress Too Much?

Stress isn't always bad. A little bit of stress can help you stay focused, energetic, and able to meet new challenges in the workplace. It's what keeps you on your toes during a presentation or alert to prevent accidents or costly mistakes. But in today's hectic world, the workplace too often seems like an emotional roller coaster. Long hours, tight deadlines, and ever-increasing demands can leave you feeling worried, drained, and overwhelmed. And when stress exceeds your ability to cope, it stops being helpful and starts causing damage to your mind and body—as well as to your job satisfaction.

If stress on the job is interfering with your work performance, health, or personal life, it's time to take action. No matter what you do for a living, or how stressful your job is, there are plenty of things you can do to reduce your overall stress levels and regain a sense of control at work.

Common causes of workplace stress include:

• Fear of being laid off

• More overtime due to staff cutbacks

• Pressure to perform to meet rising expectations but with no increase in job satisfaction

• Pressure to work at optimum levels—all the time!

• Lack of control over how you do your work

Stress At Work Warning Signs

When you feel overwhelmed at work, you lose confidence and may become angry, irritable, or withdrawn. Other signs and symptoms of excessive stress at work include:

• Feeling anxious, irritable, or depressed

• Apathy, loss of interest in work

• Problems sleeping

• Fatigue

• Trouble concentrating

• Muscle tension or headaches

• Stomach problems

• Social withdrawal

- Loss of sex drive

- Using alcohol or drugs to cope

Beat Workplace Stress By Reaching Out

Sometimes the best stress-reducer is simply sharing your stress with someone close to you. The act of talking it out and getting support and sympathy—especially face-to-face—can be a highly-effective way of blowing off steam and regaining your sense of calm. The other person doesn't have to "fix" your problems; they just need to be a good listener.

Turn to co-workers for support. Having a solid support system at work can help buffer you from the negative effects of job stress. Just remember to listen to them and offer support when they are in need as well. If you don't have a close friend at work, you can take steps to be more social with your coworkers. When you take a break, for example, instead of directing your attention to your smartphone, try engaging your colleagues.

Lean on your friends and family members. As well as increasing social contact at work, having a strong network of supportive friends and family members is extremely important to managing stress in all areas of your life. On the flip side, the lonelier and more isolated you are, the greater your vulnerability to stress.

Build new satisfying friendships. If you don't feel that you have anyone to turn to—at work or in your free time—it's never too late to build new friendships. Meet new people with common interests by taking a class or joining a club, or by volunteering your time. As well as expanding your social network, helping others—especially those who are appreciative—delivers immense pleasure and can help significantly reduce stress.

Support Your Health With Exercise And Nutrition

When you're overly focused on work, it's easy to neglect your physical health. But when you're supporting your health with good nutrition and exercise, you're stronger and more resilient to stress.

Taking care of yourself doesn't require a total lifestyle overhaul. Even small things can lift your mood, increase your energy, and make you feel like you're back in the driver's seat.

-Make time for regular exercise

Aerobic exercise—activity that raises your heart rate and makes you sweat—is a hugely effective way to lift your mood, increase energy, sharpen focus, and relax both the mind and body. Rhythmic movement—such as walking, running, dancing, drumming, etc.—is especially soothing for the nervous system. For maximum stress relief, try to get at least 30 minutes of activity on most days. If it's easier to fit into your schedule, break up the activity into two or three shorter segments.

And when stress is mounting at work, try to take a quick break and move away from the stressful situation. Take a stroll outside the workplace if possible. Physical movement can help you regain your balance.

-Make smart, stress-busting food choices

Your food choices can have a huge impact on how you feel during the work day. Eating small, frequent and healthy meals, for example, can help your body maintain an even level of blood sugar. This maintains your energy and focus, and prevents mood swings. Low blood sugar, on the other hand, can make you feel anxious and irritable, while eating too much can make you lethargic.

Minimize sugar and refined carbs. When you're stressed, you may crave sugary snacks, baked goods, or comfort foods such as pasta or French fries. But these "feel-good" foods quickly lead to a crash in mood and energy, making symptoms of stress worse, not better.

Reduce your intake of foods that can adversely affect your mood, such as caffeine, trans fats, and foods with high levels of chemical preservatives or hormones.

Eat more Omega-3 fatty acids to give your mood a boost. The best sources are fatty fish (salmon, herring, mackerel, anchovies, sardines), seaweed, flaxseed, and walnuts.

Avoid nicotine. Smoking when you're feeling stressed may seem calming, but nicotine is a powerful stimulant, leading to higher, not lower, levels of anxiety.

Drink alcohol in moderation. Alcohol may seem like it's temporarily reducing your worries, but too much can cause anxiety as it wears off and adversely affect your mood.

Don't Skimp On Sleep

You may feel like you just don't have the time get a full night's sleep. But skimping on sleep interferes with your daytime productivity, creativity, problem-solving skills, and ability to focus. The better rested you are, the better equipped you'll be to tackle your job responsibilities and cope with workplace stress.

Improve the quality of your sleep by making healthy changes to your daytime and nightly routines. For example, go to bed and get up at the same time every day, even on weekends, be smart about what you eat and drink during the day, and make adjustments to your sleep environment. Aim for eight hours a night—the amount of sleep most adults need to operate at their best.

Turn off screens one hour before bedtime. The light emitted from TV, tablets, smartphones, and computers suppresses your body's production of melatonin and can severely disrupt your sleep.

Avoid stimulating activity and stressful situations before bedtime such as catching up on work. Instead, focus on quiet, soothing activities, such as reading or listening to soft music, while keeping lights low.

Stress and shift work

Working night, early morning, or rotating shifts can impact your sleep quality, which in turn may affect productivity and performance, leaving you more vulnerable to stress.

• Adjust your sleep-wake cycle by exposing yourself to bright light when you wake up at night and using bright lamps or daylight-simulation bulbs in your workplace. Then, wear dark glasses on your journey home to block out sunlight and encourage sleepiness.

• Limit the number of night or irregular shifts you work in a row to prevent sleep deprivation from mounting up.

• Avoid frequently rotating shifts so you can maintain the same sleep schedule.

• Eliminate noise and light from your bedroom during the day. Use blackout curtains or a sleep mask, turn off the phone, and use ear plugs or a soothing sound machine to block out daytime noise.

Prioritize And Organize

When job and workplace stress threatens to overwhelm you, there are simple, practical steps you can take to regain control.

Time Management Tips For Reducing Job Stress

Create a balanced schedule. All work and no play is a recipe for burnout. Try to find a balance between work and family life, social activities and solitary pursuits, daily responsibilities and downtime.

Leave earlier in the morning. Even 10-15 minutes can make the difference between frantically rushing and having time to ease into your day. If you're always running late, set your clocks and watches fast to give yourself extra time and decrease your stress levels.

Plan regular breaks. Make sure to take short breaks throughout the day to take a walk, chat with a friendly face, or practice a relaxation technique. Also try to get away from your desk or work station for lunch. It will help you relax and recharge and be more, not less, productive.

Establish healthy boundaries. Many of us feel pressured to be available 24 hours a day or obliged to keep checking our smartphones for work-related messages and updates. But it's important to maintain periods where you're not working or thinking about work. That may mean not checking emails or taking work calls at home in the evening or on weekends.

Don't over-commit yourself. Avoid scheduling things back-to-back or trying to fit too much into one day. If you've got too much on your plate, distinguish between the "shoulds" and the "musts." Drop tasks that aren't truly necessary to the bottom of the list or eliminate them entirely.

Task Management Tips For Reducing Job Stress

Prioritize tasks. Tackle high-priority tasks first. If you have something particularly unpleasant to do, get it over with early. The rest of your day will be more pleasant as a result.

Break projects into small steps. If a large project seems overwhelming, focus on one manageable step at a time, rather than taking on everything at once.

Delegate responsibility. You don't have to do it all yourself. Let go of the desire to control every little step. You'll be letting go of unnecessary stress in the process.

Be willing to compromise. Sometimes, if you and a co-worker or boss can both adjust your expectations a little, you'll be able to find a happy middle ground that reduces the stress levels for everyone.

Break Bad Habits That Contribute To Workplace Stress

Many of us make job stress worse with negative thoughts and behavior. If you can turn these self-defeating habits around, you'll find employer-imposed stress easier to handle.

Resist perfectionism. When you set unrealistic goals for yourself, you're setting yourself up to fall short. Aim to do your best; no one can ask for more than that.

Flip your negative thinking. If you focus on the downside of every situation and interaction, you'll find yourself drained of energy and motivation. Try to think positively about your work, avoid negative co-workers, and pat yourself on the back about small accomplishments, even if no one else does.

Don't try to control the uncontrollable. Many things at work are beyond our control, particularly the behavior of other people. Rather than stressing out over them, focus on the things you can control, such as the way you choose to react to problems.

Look for humor in the situation. When used appropriately, humor is a great way to relieve stress in the workplace. When you or those around you start taking work too seriously, find a way to lighten the mood by sharing a joke or funny story.

Clean up your act. If your desk or work space is a mess, file and throw away the clutter; just knowing where everything is can save time and reduce stress.

Be Proactive About Your Job And Your Workplace Duties

When we feel uncertain, helpless, or out of control, our stress levels are the highest. Here are some things you can do to regain a sense of control over your job and career.

Talk to your employer about workplace stressors. Healthy and happy employees are more productive, so your employer has an incentive to tackle workplace stress whenever possible. Rather than rattling off a list of complaints, let your employer know about specific conditions that are impacting your work performance.

Clarify your job description. Ask your supervisor for an updated description of your job duties and responsibilities. You may find that some of the tasks that have piled up are not included in your job description, and you can gain a little leverage by pointing out that you've been putting in work over and above the parameters of your job.

Request a transfer. If your workplace is large enough, you might be able to escape a toxic environment by transferring to another department.

Ask for new duties. If you've been doing the exact same work for a long time, ask to try something new: a different grade level, a different sales territory, a different machine.

Take time off. If burnout seems inevitable, take a complete break from work. Go on vacation, use up your sick days, ask for a temporary leave-of-absence—anything to remove yourself from the situation. Use the time away to recharge your batteries and gain perspective.

Look For Satisfaction And Meaning In Your Work

Feeling bored or unsatisfied with how you spend most of the workday can cause high levels of stress and take a serious toll on your physical and mental health. But for many of us, having a dream job that we find meaningful and rewarding is just that: a dream. Even if you're not in a position to look for another career that you love and are passionate about—and most of us aren't—you can still find purpose and joy in a job that you don't love.

Even in some mundane jobs, you can often focus on how your contributions help others, for example, or provide a much-needed product or service. Focus on aspects of the job that you do enjoy, even if it's just chatting with your coworkers at lunch. Changing your attitude towards your job can also help you regain a sense of purpose and control.

How Managers Or Employers Can Reduce Stress At Work

Employees who are suffering from work-related stress can lead to lower productivity, lost workdays, and a higher turnover of staff. As a manager, supervisor, or employer though, you can help lower workplace stress. The first step is to act as a positive role model. If you can remain calm in stressful situations, it's much easier for your employees to follow suit.

Consult your employees. Talk to them about the specific factors that make their jobs stressful. Some things, such as failing equipment, understaffing, or a lack of supervisor feedback may be relatively straightforward to address. Sharing information with employees can also reduce uncertainty about their jobs and futures.

Communicate with your employees one-on-one. Listening attentively face-to-face will make an employee feel heard and understood. This will help lower their stress and yours, even if you're unable to change the situation.

Deal with workplace conflicts in a positive way. Respect the dignity of each employee; establish a zero-tolerance policy for harassment.

Give workers opportunities to participate in decisions that affect their jobs. Get employee input on work rules, for example. If they're involved in the process, they'll be more committed.

Avoid unrealistic deadlines. Make sure the workload is suitable to your employees' abilities and resources.

Clarify your expectations. Clearly define employees' roles, responsibilities, and goals. Make sure management actions are fair and consistent with organizational values.

Offer rewards and incentives. Praise work accomplishments verbally and organization-wide. Schedule potentially stressful periods followed by periods of fewer tight deadlines. Provide opportunities for social interaction among employees.

Chapter 19: Common Mistakes People Make When Dealing With Stress

There are some very common mistakes one is likely to make as they strive to manage stress. These are normally the very same things that slow their process of recovery, or make it difficult altogether. It is a good idea for you to learn of these mistakes and avoid them putting yourself a step ahead on the road to recovery. Let's therefore get to know each of them:

Refusing Help

There are those who refuse help from family and friends just because they feel ashamed, or have allowed their feelings of anger or irritability to be in complete control. This is normally a huge mistake, as it prevents you from finding the right help or support you require. When you don't want your loved ones to be by your side, then the healing will take longer than imagined.

Making Rushed Decisions

You could also be tempted to make rushed decisions and this is never advisable, especially with your state of mind. Most times, you are not yourself, and are being guided by negative thoughts, sadness and anger that you feel inside. Always take time or have someone close to you to help you through any kind of decision making process. If you don't, then you might make decisions that end up having negative effects in the future and this will be a source of more stress.

Procrastination

It is also a mistake for someone with stress to keep procrastinating responsibilities just because you are not in the mood. The more you pile-on tasks the more challenging they become for you to accomplish them. This makes for a cluttered mind and environment and it will also contribute to increased stress levels.

Ignoring Stress and Its Symptoms

Stress is something that should never be ignored, because it doesn't easily go away on its own. What it does is keep growing inside you and at the end of it all it does more damage to your general health. This is why we are always advised to be in touch with our lives, and to notice any kind of changes. With the idea in mind of what stress is and its symptoms, you should always take action when you notice it growing in you.

Eating Habits

The most common signs of a person with stress is that there is always a change in eating habits. You will need to be very keen when managing stress and make sure that you don't over-eat or under-eat as this will impact on your general health and the results will be very negative. What happens when you realize you have gained so much weight or have lost so much, your worry makes your stress levels increase so whether under stress or not you should watch what you eat and how much you eat.

Being Cruel To People around You

I understand that it is your stress levels that are making you feel angry or irritated every other time, but try and not allow those feelings affect your relationships. Some people may not be very understanding, and what will happen when everyone starts rejecting you? Your life starts becoming more and more miserable, and the stress will keep prevailing.

Chapter 20: How To Manage Stress At Work?

The ability to manage stress in an effective way is very important to live a balanced life. The following techniques will help you to relief stress.

Stress, the body's reaction towards stressful situations, is a state of mental suspense that can have negative influences on our lives and on our health. Stress management helps you to reduce the negative side-effects of stress and allows you to handle stressful situations calmer than before.

In short: it helps you to improve your ability to cope with stress and to avoid stress related conditions, such as chronic headaches, heart diseases and depression. Another benefit of stress management techniques is that it will help you to avoid careless mistakes, which would cost you a lot of time in order to cut out these mistakes.

How to manage stress at the workplace?

Many employees consider stress as an essential part at their workplace that helps them to meet deadlines and increases their productivity. However, when stress becomes chronic it is important to take counter-measures.

Time Management:

Time management is an essential skill when it comes to the ability to reduce stress. In fact: improper time management can be one of the main reasons that cause stress, as we might not be able to meet deadlines and can't accomplish the targeted tasks and goals.

In our corporate world we are facing workload and time limitations nearly every day, which makes it essential to apply effective time management techniques.

Physical Activity:

Physical activity and regular exercise can help you to relief stress in an effective way. Sport in general increases the productions of endorphins and decreases stress hormones.

You do not necessarily need to join a gym or start running every morning; you can also make use of the stress relieving effect of physical activity at the workplace.

As a rule of thumb: keep your body moving. Instead of taking the elevator you could walk up the staircases, take a stroll during your lunch break or just stretch your body in a regular interval, which sitting on your office chair.

Organization

Start prioritizing your tasks from A - very important to C - unimportant and organize your tasks accordingly to their importance and urgency.

If a task is very important and urgent you should focus your time and energy towards the accomplishment of this task, rather than a task that is important but not urgent at all. I would recommend you to invest five minutes before starting to work where you create a to-do-list with all your upcoming tasks and their prioritization.

Conclusion

Stress is a major cause of burnout. Stress may cause serious health conditions, which may trigger death in rare situations. Stress management strategies have been proven to have a beneficial impact on stress mitigation. Strategies are intended for encouragement, so readers can seek recommendations from sufficiently trained health providers whether they have questions regarding stress-related illnesses or are experiencing stress triggers causing serious unhappiness. Additionally, it is important to seek the advice of health care professionals before making significant adjustments in nutrition or activity.

Heart attacks, cancer, and various other syndromes like the issues of the digestive tract, skin conditions, colds, headaches, pains, bronchial issues or asthma, strokes, and others, have all been connected to stress. After taking a look at how stress impacted me and observing how it influenced those around me, I began devising and implementing certain alternative techniques in my day-to- day life with a view of reducing my stress levels.

When the body is under stress, it starts generating specific hormones in an attempt to recover equilibrium. These hormones help us take essential steps to lower stress levels and are generally referred to as 'fight or flight' hormones that are triggered in the presence of a threat. They prompt us that we should either fight the problem or run from the threat.

Physical signs or manifestations of the stress we experience are negative changes in the rhythm of our heartbeat. This increases blood circulation around our bodies and also muscle mass as it prepares us for the obstacle of what exists ahead, and also while our body is going through this stress, we also experience loss of appetite. Additionally, stress takes a toll on our immune systems, making us more susceptible to getting sick. The fight or flight sensation we experience is certainly an essential mechanism for our survival and was more so during the time of our ancestors when they had to run from real life predators. Yet, over the generations, as we have evolved and no longer have to run from animals trying to kill us, this mechanism fight or flight reaction is triggered when our mother in law upsets

us, traffic is backed up, a looming deadline approaches etc - and this reaction that once helped protect us from predators now hurts us by releasing too much stress hormone whenever we face stress - and the kind that is not going to cause imminent danger.

Trying to manage all the many facets of your life is undoubtedly the primary cause of remuneration. You are doomed if you feverishly worry over every small detail about each thing you should do in every minute of your life in fear of what might occur in the next moment.... The very best thing you can do for yourself is to learn how to calm down, slow down, get grounded, learn how to be present in each moment and live that moment - not ahead into the future or back in the past. The universe has your back, so you need to relax and make the most of every moment - be here now.

At the end of the day, understand that each of us holds the potential to attain whatever we have dreamed of, and the only thing we have to do is to steer ourselves in the right direction, be calm and present and do our best to eliminate our deterrents. And that makes all the difference!

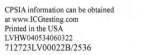